THE
SIMULATED ADMINISTRATIVE MEDICAL OFFICE

Practicum Skills for Medical Assistants

powered by  SimChart®
for the medical office

THE SIMULATED ADMINISTRATIVE MEDICAL OFFICE

Practicum Skills for Medical Assistants

2nd Edition

powered by **SimChart®**
for the medical office

JULIE PEPPER, CMA (AAMA), BS

Program Director
Health Navigator Program
Instructor
Medical Assisting Program
Chippewa Valley Technical College
Eau Claire, Wisconsin

ELSEVIER

Elsevier
3251 Riverport Lane
St. Louis, Missouri 63043

THE SIMULATED ADMINISTRATIVE MEDICAL OFFICE, 2e   ISBN: 978-0-323-82951-9

Notice

Practitioners and researchers must always rely on their own experience and knowledge in evaluating and using any information, methods, compounds or experiments described herein. Because of rapid advances in the medical sciences, in particular, independent verification of diagnoses and drug dosages should be made. To the fullest extent of the law, no responsibility is assumed by Elsevier, authors, editors or contributors for any injury and/or damage to persons or property as a matter of products liability, negligence or otherwise, or from any use or operation of any methods, products, instructions, or ideas contained in the material herein.

Previous editions copyrighted 2015.

International Standard Book Number: 978-0-323-82951-9

Content Strategist: Kristin Wilhelm
Senior Content Development Specialist: Priyadarshini Pandey
Publishing Services Manager: Deepthi Unni
Project Manager: Sindhuraj Thulasingam
Design Direction: Bridget Hoette

Printed in India

Last digit is the print number: 9   8   7   6   5   4   3   2   1

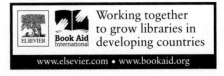

I would not be in the position to write this book if a dear friend had not told me about the medical assisting profession so many years ago. That conversation put me on this path. What a journey it has been, all thanks to Jill Lawrence!

I would like to thank the team at Elsevier for putting their trust in me again for this edition. It has been a joy to work with Kristin R. Wilhelm, Priyadarshini Pandey, Bridget Hoette, and Sindhuraj Thulasingam.

I could not have completed this work without the support of my family, Jeff, Megan, Jon, and Callie. You have been amazing throughout this whole process. I could not ask for more encouraging and patient people with whom to share all of this.

In memory of my mom, who was always so proud of my accomplishments.

Preface

In all healthcare professions, there is a need to have an understanding of how electronic health records (EHRs) function. This book was written to address how the EHR functions in the administrative area of a medical clinic. It will take students on a 10-day journey of accomplishing tasks that are vital to the success of a medical clinic.

The purpose of *The Simulated Administrative Medical Office* is to simulate the tasks that an administrative medical assistant would perform while working in a medical practice. The student will complete tasks related to appointment scheduling, completion of common forms, inventory, correspondence, telephone messages, scribing, and coding and billing.

This textbook uses SimChart for the Medical Office (sold separately) as the basis for the practicum experience. The software allows students to become familiar with the functionality of an EHR. The skills learned while accomplishing those tasks will be transferable to whichever EHR software students encounter in the real world. The tasks will help to build students' confidence in their abilities to use any EHR software.

SimChart for the Medical Office is web-based software that allows for instructor and student flexibility. Students can access the software wherever there is a computer and a connection to the Internet. Instructors can use the software for face-to-face classes, hybrid classes, or completely online classes.

If you do not already have access to SimChart for the Medical Office, contact your Elsevier Educational Solutions Consultant for purchase options.

Organization

The tasks of this text are organized over 10 days to simulate a 2-week practicum experience. Each day consists of 10 tasks that a medical assistant might be called on to perform during a day in an internship or practicum. The tasks begin simply and then build on each other, gaining in complexity as familiarity with SimChart for the Medical Office is achieved.

New to This Edition

- Twice the number of tasks that increase in complexity throughout the day and week.
- Text discussions to provide context for on-the-job reference, especially on insurance and coding.
- Illustrations that include realistic patient forms and screen shots.

Distinctive Features

- 100 *SimChart for the Medical Office* tasks organized into 2 weeks of work, each simulating actual office duties, providing practice with patient scheduling, billing, insurance processing, and more.
- Case-based format that applies all tasks to realistic patient encounters, building critical thinking and problem-solving skills.
- Step-by-step instructions to simplify the tasks, helping you learn accuracy and speed within a fast-paced medical office.
- Online forms and documents simulate the office experience and support the electronic workflow.
- SimChart for the Medical Office screenshots throughout to help you follow along easily
- Alignment with ABHES and CAAHEP competencies for Medical Assisting.
- Content that supports preparation for certification as a Medical Assistant and Certified Electronic Health Records Specialist.

For the Student

- Audio clips of patient messages to provide a realistic simulation of checking and responding to messages in a medical office.
- Other forms and documents to assist students with their daily front office duties.

For the Instructor

- Image collection of SimChart for the Medical Office screenshots.
- Solutions to the daily tasks to provide guidance on what the student work should look like when completed in the EHR exercises.
- Commission on Accreditation of Allied Health Education Programs (CAAHEP), Accrediting Bureau of Health Education Schools (ABHES), and Certified Electronic Health Records Specialist (CEHRS) correlation grids to show how each task is tied to the standards of the field.

Contents

1. Day One

Task 1.1 Prepare the Scheduling Matrix

For your first day at your practicum at the Walden-Martin Family Medical Clinic, Jill, your mentor, wants you to get familiar with how the appointment schedule works. The appointment schedule is the basis for how the whole medical office functions (Fig. 1.1). Knowing how to use the electronic schedule will make you a valuable asset to any medical office.

The first step in creating a workable schedule is determining the length of the shortest visit type, such as a follow-up or recheck appointment for an established patient. Typically this would be 10–15 minutes. The matrix would then be set up with 10- or 15-minute time slots. For more comprehensive visits, such as a new patient examination or complete physical examination, multiple time slots would be used. These visits are typically 30–45 minutes. For those visits three, time slots would be utilized. Walden-Martin Family Medical Clinic has determined that the shortest visit would be 15 minutes. Box 1.1 shows the timeframe for the various encounter types found in SimChart for the Medical Office.

The next step would be blocking out times for which the providers are not available. There are times when all providers are not available to see patients, such as a monthly staff meeting, but there are also times that each individual provider would not be available. It is important that the matrix is set up correctly so that everyone knows which times are available for patients to be seen.

Your first task is to prepare the schedule for the next 6 months by blocking off times when the physicians will not be available for appointments. You will be blocking off times for the providers, including lunch breaks, hospital and nursing home rounds, vacation times, and conferences.

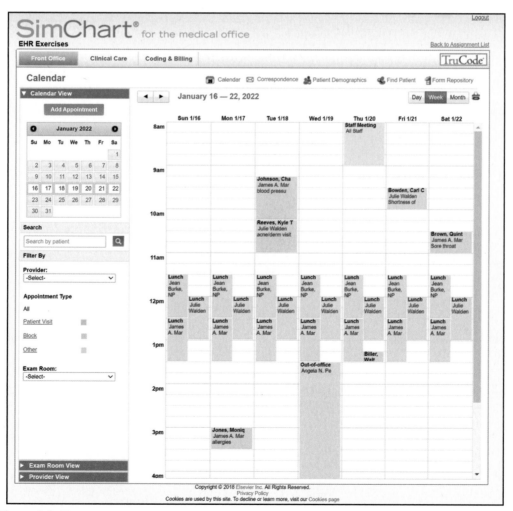

Figure 1.1 The appointment schedule.

James A. Martin, MD, Schedule

Lunch. Dr. Martin takes his lunch break daily from 12:30 to 1:30 PM.

1. Click the **EHR Exercises** button to enter the simulation (Fig. 1.2).
2. Click the **Add Appointment** button. Note that all fields with an asterisk (*) are mandatory. You must have an entry in those fields in order to move forward.
3. In the **Appointment Type** field, select the **Block** radio button.
4. In the **Block Type** field, select **Lunch** from the drop-down menu.
5. In the **For** field, select **James A. Martin, MD** from the drop-down menu.
6. In the **Date** field, select today's date using the calendar picker.
7. Select a **Start Time** of **12:30 PM** and an **End Time** of **01:30 PM** from the drop-down menus.
8. This is an appointment that will be occurring every day, so the **Recurrence** box needs to be checked. In the **Recurrence Pattern** field, select the **Daily** radio button. In the **Recurrence Duration** field, use the calendar picker to select the **End By** radio button and choose the date that is 6 months from today's date.
9. Click the **Save** button. You may receive a message stating "New appointment conflicts with an existing appointment." Click the **OK** button. You will be rescheduling those appointments in a future task. You will see a confirmation message; click the **OK** button.

Hospital Rounds. Dr. Martin does rounds at the hospital daily from 8:00 to 9:00 AM.

1. Click the **Add Appointment** button.
2. In the **Appointment Type** field, select the **Block** radio button.

BOX 1.1

Appropriate Appointment Times for Patients

Visit Type	Length of Visit
Annual exam	45 minutes
Comprehensive visit	30 minutes
Follow-up/established visit	15 minutes
New patient visit	45 minutes
Urgent visit	30 minutes
Wellness exam	30 minutes
6-month visit	15 minutes

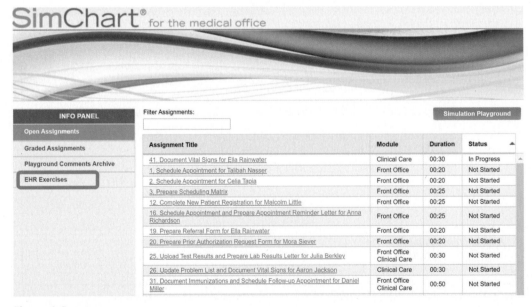

Figure 1.2 EHR exercises.

3. In the **Block Type** field, select **Other** from the drop-down menu and enter "Rounds" in the **Other** textbox.
4. In the **For** field, select **James A. Martin, MD** from the drop-down menu.
5. In the **Date** field, select today's date, using the calendar picker.
6. Select a **Start Time** of **08:00 AM** and an **End Time** of **09:00 AM** from the drop-down menus.
7. This appointment will be occurring every day, so select the **Recurrence** box. In the **Recurrence Duration** field, select the **End By** radio button and choose the date that is 6 months from today's date using the calendar picker.
8. Click the **Save** button.

Nursing Home Rounds. Dr. Martin makes rounds at the nursing home from 1:30 to 5:00 PM on Wednesdays.

1. Click the **Add Appointment** button.
2. In the **Appointment Type** field, select the **Block** radio button.
3. In the **Block Type** field, select **Other** from the drop-down menu and enter "Nursing Home Rounds" in the **Other** textbox.
4. In the **For** field, select **James A. Martin, MD** from the drop-down menu.
5. In the **Date** field, select the next Wednesday using the calendar picker.
6. Select a **Start Time** of **01:30 PM** and an **End Time** of **5:00 PM** from the drop-down menus.
7. This appointment will be occurring once a week, so select the **Recurrence** box. In the **Recurrence Duration** field, select the **End By** radio button and choose the date that is 6 months from today's date, using the calendar picker.
8. Click the **Save** button.

Vacation. Dr. Martin will be taking vacation for the first full week of next month. He will be gone Monday through Friday.

1. Click the **Add Appointment** button.
2. In the **Appointment Type** field, select the **Block** radio button.
3. In the **Block Type** field, select **Out-of-office** from the drop-down menu.
4. In the **For** field, select **James A. Martin, MD** from the drop-down menu.
5. In the **Date** field, select the Monday of the first full week of the next month using the calendar picker.
6. Select a **Start Time** of **08:00 AM** and an **End Time** of **06:00 PM** from the drop-down menus.
7. This appointment will be occurring daily, so select the **Recurrence** box.
8. In the **Recurrence Pattern** field, select the **Daily** radio button.
9. In the **Recurrence Duration** field, select the **End By** radio button and choose the Friday of the week of this vacation, using the calendar picker.
10. Click the **Save** button.

Conference. Dr. Martin will be attending a full-day conference on innovations in diabetes treatments next Tuesday.

1. Click the **Add Appointment** button.
2. In the **Appointment Type** field, select the **Block** radio button.
3. In the **Block Type** field, select **Out-of-office** from the drop-down menu.
4. In the **For** field, select **James A. Martin, MD** from the drop-down menu.
5. In the **Date** field, select next Tuesday using the calendar picker.
6. Select a **Start Time** of **08:00 AM** and an **End Time** of **06:00 PM** from the drop-down menus.
7. Click the **Save** button.

You have now successfully set up the appointment matrix for Dr. Martin. Using the process you have learned, set up the appointment matrix for Dr. Julie Walden and Jean Burke, NP, using the information provided below.

Julie Walden, MD, Schedule

1. Lunch break daily from 12:00 to 1:00 PM.
2. Hospital rounds daily from 8:30 to 9:30 AM.
3. Nursing home rounds weekly on Thursdays from 1:00 to 4:00 PM.
4. She will be taking vacation the second week of next month and will be gone Monday to Friday.
5. She will be presenting at the AAMA conference 2 weeks from today at 1:00 PM and will be gone for the afternoon.

Jean Burke, NP, Schedule

1. Lunch break daily from 11:30 AM to 12:30 PM.
2. Hospital rounds daily from 3:30 to 4:30 PM.
3. She will be taking vacation 3 weeks from Monday and will be gone Monday to Friday.

The appointment matrix is now in place and now you can schedule appointments for patients. Jill lets you observe how she handles this, and now it is your turn to schedule appointments for an established patient. During your observation, you notice that Jill was able to access the new appointment window by clicking within the appointment calendar. You can either use this method or click the Add Appointment button to complete the task below.

Task 1.2 Reschedule Appointments

Jill reminds you that when you were setting up the appointment matrix, you received a notification that the new appointment (lunch, rounds, vacation, etc.) conflicted with an existing appointment. You now need to reschedule those patient appointments that conflict with the newly established matrix.

James A. Martin, MD, Schedule

1. To view Dr. Martin's schedule, select **James A. Martin, MD** from the **Provider** drop-down menu in the Calendar View section of the information panel on the left side of the screen (Fig. 1.3). Now the calendar will show only Dr. Martin's schedule.
2. Locate the patient appointments, shown in blue, that are scheduled at the same time as the blocked appointments, shown in pink.
3. Click on the patient appointment to view the details of that appointment. If this is a reccurring appointment, you will be asked if you want to "Open this occurrence" or "Open the series."
4. Select the radio button next to **Open the Series** and then click the **OK** button. This will change all appointments scheduled at that time for this patient.
5. Adjust the start time and end time so that the appointment no longer conflicts with the blocked appointment (e.g., on the 5th of the month, Quinton Brown has a 30-minute recurring appointment scheduled at 8:30 AM. This now conflicts with Dr. Martin's rounds. The new start time should be 9:00 AM, and the new end time should be 9:30 AM). Click the **Save** button.
6. You will see a confirmation message. Click the **OK** button. Continue to review the calendar and reschedule the appointments as necessary, using the steps above.

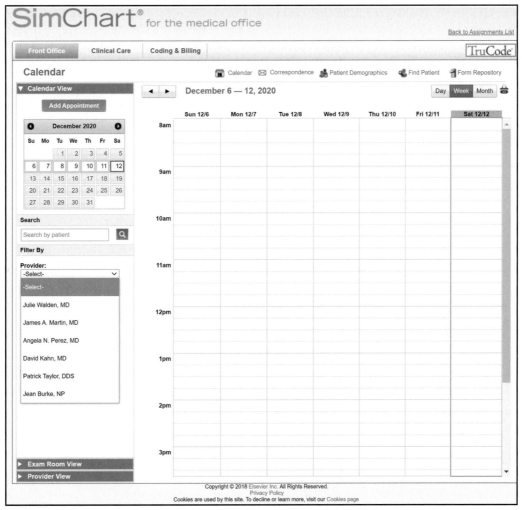

Figure 1.3 Dr. Martin's schedule.

Julie Walden, MD, Schedule

1. To view Dr. Walden's schedule, select **Julie Walden, MD** from the Provider drop-down menu in the Calendar View section of the information panel on the left side of the screen. Now the calendar will show only Dr. Walden's schedule.
2. Locate the patient appointments, shown in blue, that are scheduled at the same time as the blocked appointments, shown in pink.
3. Review the calendar and reschedule the appointments as necessary.

Jean Burke, NP, Schedule

1. To view Jean Burke's schedule, select **Jean Burke, NP** from the Provider drop-down menu in the Calendar View section of the information panel on the left side of the screen. Now the calendar will show only Jean's schedule.
2. Locate the patient appointments, shown in blue, that are scheduled at the same time as the blocked appointments, shown in pink.
3. Review the calendar and reschedule the appointments as necessary.

Scheduling Patient Appointments

When scheduling appointments for patients, it is important to keep in mind the length of time for each type of appointment. When talking with the patient, you will determine what type of appointment is needed. The reason for the visit is called the chief complaint. That will determine when the appointment should be scheduled, and the chief complaint is documented for that appointment. If the patient is being seen because they are ill, the signs/and symptoms should be documented. Annual exams and wellness exams are done once a year. You may need to look at the patient's health record to determine when they were last in. Many insurance companies will not pay for an annual exam if it is done before 365 days have passed. Follow-up visits should be scheduled based on the provider's order.

Offering patients some choices of date and time can help to ensure that the patient keeps the appointment. You can explain that the doctor would like the appointment to be in a week (e.g., for a follow-up exam) and then ask if Tuesday or Wednesday would be better. After the day has been determined, ask if they would like a morning or afternoon appointment. You can then offer that patient the time that is open in the provider's schedule.

Tasks 1.3, 1.4, and 1.5 will give you practice in scheduling appointments for established patients.

Task 1.3 Schedule a Follow-up Appointment for an Established Patient

Al Neviaser, DOB 06/21/1968, is an established patient of Dr. Martin. He has called in to schedule an appointment to have his blood pressure checked. This will be a follow-up visit that is 15 minutes in length (Box 1.1). The patient has requested that this appointment be on a Friday during his lunch time, between 11:30 AM and 12:30 PM.

Established Patient Visit

1. Click the **Add Appointment** button or click within the appointment calendar.
2. In the **Appointment Type** field, select the **Patient Visit** radio button.
3. In the **Visit Type** field, select **Follow-up/Established Visit** from the drop-down menu.
4. In the **Chief Complaint** field, enter "Blood pressure check."
5. Select the **Search Existing Patients** radio button.

 PROFESSIONALISM

It is always a good idea to search existing patient records, even if the patient has stated that he or she is a new patient. This reduces the risk of creating duplicate records for patients.

6. Enter "Neviaser" in the **Last Name** field and click the **Go** button.
7. Verify the DOB, select the radio button next to his name, and click the **Select** button.
8. In the **Date** field, select Friday's date, using the calendar picker.
9. Select a **Start Time** of **12:00 PM** and an **End Time** of **12:15 PM** from the drop-down menus.
10. Click the **Save** button. You will see a confirmation message.
11. Click the **OK** button. The appointment will appear on the calendar.

Task 1.4 Schedule an Urgent Appointment for an Established Patient

Patients schedule visits for a variety of reasons, and most can wait at least a day or two, but an urgent visit is used when a patient needs to be seen on the same day. An urgent visit would be scheduled when a patient has a problem that requires prompt attention but is not life-threatening (which would be considered an emergency). If the situation is an emergency, the provider often instructs the patient to go straight to the closest hospital emergency department instead of the office. Many healthcare organizations leave open time slots on the daily schedule to accommodate urgent visits. Some reasons for an urgent visit include:

- Vomiting or persistent diarrhea
- Wheezing or shortness of breath
- Abdominal pain
- Animal bite
- An adult patient with a fever over 102 °F
- Small cuts that may need sutures
- Sprains and strains
- Dehydration

Noemi Rodriquez, DOB 11/04/1971, is an established patient of Jean Burke, NP. She has called in stating that she has had a temperature of 102.8 °F for the last 2 days along with vomiting and diarrhea. She is concerned about how poorly she is feeling and would like to come in to see Jean Burke. Schedule an Urgent Visit (see Box 1.1 for the length of time needed for this visit). Noemi states that her husband will be home at noon and requests that the appointment be after that time so he can drive.

Using the process learned in Task 1.3 schedule an Urgent Visit for Noemi Rodriquez with Jean Burke, NP. Remember that documenting the chief complaint is part of scheduling the appointment.

Task 1.5 Schedule a Wellness Exam Appointment for an Established Patient

A wellness exam is most often associated with Medicare beneficiaries. Medicare pays for an annual wellness visit for people covered by Medicare. This is different from an annual exam. A wellness exam is less comprehensive than annual physical examination. During a wellness exam, the patient works with the provider to develop or update a personalized prevention plan to help prevent disease and disability. A Health Risk Assessment form will be completed and reviewed to help develop the best personalized plan to keep the patient healthy. Along with reviewing the Health Risk Assessment form, there will be a review of medical and family history; review of medications; height, weight, and blood pressure will be taken; a cognitive impairment assessment may be done; and advance care planning maybe discussed.

Robert Caudill, DOB 10/31/1940, is calling to schedule his wellness exam. You have reviewed is records and see that he has Medicare for insurance and that his last wellness exam was more than a year ago. Mr. Caudill states that he meets with a group of his old high school classmates for breakfast Thursday mornings, but he would be available any other day of the week and he has no time of day preference (see Box 1.1 for the length of time needed for this visit).

1. Using the process learned in Task 1.3, schedule a wellness exam visit for Robert Caudill with Jean Burke, NP. See Box 1.1 for the length of time needed for this visit.

Scheduling and Registering New Patients

Now that you have experience in scheduling an appointment for established patients, Jill would like you to schedule new patient appointments, which require a bit more information. When scheduling an appointment for a new patient, some basic demographic information is obtained over the telephone; more complete information for registration is obtained when the patient comes in for the appointment.

Tasks 1.6, 1.7, 1.8, and 1.9 will give you practice in scheduling and registering new patients.

Task 1.6 Schedule a New Adult Patient Appointment

Angela Moore calls the clinic and would like to schedule an appointment with Dr. Walden. She states, "I have an itchy rash that's getting worse." According to the medical office's procedures, this type of complaint should be seen on the same day. A new patient visit is scheduled for 45 minutes (Box 1.1).

New Adult Patient Visit

1. Open Dr. Walden's schedule.
2. Find the first available 45-minute appointment for today and click on that time slot.
3. In the **Appointment Type** field, select the **Patient Visit** radio button.
4. In the **Visit Type** field, select **New Patient Visit** from the drop-down menu.
5. In the **Chief Complaint** field, enter "Itchy rash."
6. Select the **Search Existing Patients** radio button.
7. Enter "Moore" in the **Last Name** field and click the **Go** button.
8. If the patient's name does not exist in the system, click the **Cancel** button. A confirmation message will appear. Click the **OK** button.
9. Select the **Create New Patient** radio button.
10. Enter "Moore" in the **Last Name** field and "Angela" in the **First Name** field.
11. Using the calendar picker, enter 10/25/1992 in the **Date of Birth** field. The **Age** field will autopopulate.
12. Select the radio button next to **Female**.
13. Enter "123-828-1886" in the **Home Phone** field.
14. Select **Julie Walden, MD** from the **Provider** drop-down menu.
15. Angela has given you her insurance information from her insurance card (Fig. 1.4) and tells you that her SSN is 989-45-8888. Enter her insurance information and click the **Save** button. A confirmation message will appear. Click the **OK** button.
16. The **New Appointment** window will open and auto populate with some of the information you just entered.
17. Use the calendar picker to choose today's date in the **Date** field.
18. Use the drop-down menu to choose the **Start Time**.
19. Use the drop-down menu to choose an **End Time** that is 45 minutes after the start time.
20. Click the **Save** button. You will see a confirmation message. Click the **OK** button. The appointment will appear on the calendar.

When new patients arrive at the medical office, they are asked to provide more complete patient demographic information than what was obtained over the phone. They will complete a Patient Information Form to provide that information. Angela Moore has just arrived at the medical office and has completed her Patient Information Form (Fig. 1.4). You will need to enter the rest of her demographic information into the electronic health record.

Checking in Angela Moore

1. Click the **Patient Demographics** icon.
2. Enter "Moore" in the **Last Name** field and click the **Search Existing Patients** button.
3. Angela's name should appear in blue. Click on **Angela**. There are three tabs for patient demographic information: **Patient, Guarantor,** and **Insurance**. All three have mandatory fields. Complete all of the mandatory fields (*) on the **Patient** tab and enter any other information that is supplied on the Patient Information Form.
4. Click on the **Guarantor** tab, complete all mandatory fields, and enter any other information that is supplied on the Patient Information Form.
5. Click on the **Insurance** tab, complete all mandatory fields, and enter any other information that is supplied on the Patient Information Form.
6. Click on the **Save Patient** button. You will see a confirmation message. Click the **Yes** button.

WALDEN-MARTIN
FAMILY MEDICAL CLINIC
1234 ANYSTREET | ANYTOWN, ANYSTATE 12345
PHONE 123-123-1234 | FAX 123-123-5678

PATIENT INFORMATION

First Name	MI	Last Name		Date of Birth	Sex
Angela	M.	Moore		10/25/1992	F

SSN	Home Phone	Work Phone		Cell
989-45-8888	123-828-1886			

Home Address	City	State	Zip
	Anytown	AL	12345-1222

Marital Status	Employer	Driver's License #
Single	Student	

Emergency Contact	Relationship to Patient	Phone Number
Ruth Moore		

RESPONSIBLE PARTY INFORMATION   SELF ☐

First Name	MI	Last Name		Date of Birth	Sex
Julie	MD	Walden			

SSN	Home Phone	Work Phone		Cell
		123-552-9057		

Home Address	City	State	Zip
1234 Anystreet	Anytown	AL	12345

Employer		Relationship to Patient
Morgan's Office Supply		Self

INSURANCE INFORMATION

Primary Insurance Carrier	Phone Number
Aetna	1-800-123-2222

Address	City	State	Zip
1234 Insurance Way	Anytown	AL	12345

Policy Holder Name (if different from patient)	Phone	Date of Birth	Sex
Angela Moore	123-251-9686		

Policy Number	Group Number
654123789	WM 753

Secondary Insurance Carrier	Phone Number

Address	City	State	Zip

Policy Holder Name (if different from patient)	Phone	Date of Birth	Sex

Policy Number	Group Number

I hereby give lifetime authorization for payment of insurance benefits to be made directly to Walden-Martin Medical Group, and any assisting physicians, for services rendered. I understand that I am financially responsible for all charges whether or not they are covered by insurance. In the event of default, I agree to pay all costs of collection, and reasonable attorney's fees. I hereby authorize this healthcare provider to release all information necessary to secure the payment of benefits. I further agree that a photocopy of this agreement shall be as valid as the original.

Signature _Angela Moore_	Date

AETNA   1234 Insurance Way

MEMBER NAME: Moore, Angela

POLICY #: 654123789

GROUP #: WM753   **EFFECTIVE DATE:** 02/15/2022

CO-PAY: $25   DRUG CO-PAY
SPECIALIST CO-PAY: $35   GENERIC: $10
XRAY/LAB BENEFIT: $250   NAME BRAND: $50

CLAIMS/INQUIRIES: 1-800-123-2222

Figure 1.4 Patient information form and insurance card for Angela Moore.

James Brown has just moved to town with his daughter. It is time for her annual examination and he would like to get her established with Angela Perez, MD. Mr. Brown doesn't work on Wednesdays and would like an appointment early in the day on the next available Wednesday.

1. Open Dr. Perez's schedule.
2. Find the first available 45-minute appointment on a Wednesday morning and click on that time slot.
3. In the **Appointment Type** field, select the **Patient Visit** radio button.
4. In the **Visit Type** field, select **New Patient Visit** from the drop-down menu.
5. In the **Chief Complaint** field, enter "Annual exam."
6. Select the **Search Existing Patients** radio button.
7. Enter "Brown" in the **Last Name** field and click the **Go** button.
8. If the patient's name does not exist in the system, click the **Cancel** button. A confirmation message will appear. Click the **OK** button.
9. Select the **Create New Patient** radio button.
10. Enter "Brown" in the **Last Name** field and "Christina" in the **First Name** field.
11. Using the calendar picker, enter 08/03/2017 in the **Date of Birth** field. The **Age** field will auto populate.
12. Select the radio button next to **Female**.
13. Enter "123-521-9686" in the **Home Phone** field.
14. Select **Angela Perez, MD** from the **Provider** drop-down menu.
15. James has given you the insurance information from his insurance card (Fig. 1.5) and tells you that his SSN is 869-50-5420. Enter the insurance information and click the **Save** button. A confirmation message will appear. Click the **OK** button.
16. The **New Appointment** window will open and auto populate with some of the information you just entered.
17. Use the drop-down menu to choose the **Start Time**.
18. Use the drop-down menu to choose an **End Time** that is 45 minutes after the start time.
19. Click the **Save** button. You will see a confirmation message. Click the **OK** button. The appointment will appear on the calendar.

WALDEN-MARTIN
FAMILY MEDICAL CLINIC
1234 ANYSTREET | ANYTOWN, ANYSTATE 12345
PHONE 123-123-1234 | FAX 123-123-5678

JULIE WALDEN MD
JAMES MARTIN MD
DAVID KAHN MD
ANGELA PEREZ MD
PATRICK TAYLOR DDS
JEAN BURKE NP

PATIENT INFORMATION

First Name	MI	Last Name		Date of Birth	Sex
Christina		Brown		8/3/2001	F

SSN	Home Phone	Work Phone		Cell
503-18-1456	123-521-9686			

Home Address	City		State	Zip
89 Collins Way	Anytown		AL	12345-1234

Marital Status	Employer	Driver's License #
Single	Student	

Emergency Contact	Relationship to Patient	Phone Number
Mary Brown	Mother	123-251-9686

RESPONSIBLE PARTY INFORMATION   SELF ☐

First Name	MI	Last Name		Date of Birth	Sex
James		Brown		10/5/1975	M

SSN	Home Phone	Work Phone		Cell
869-50-5420	123-251-9686			

Home Address	City		State	Zip
89 Collins Way	Anytown		AL	12345-1234

Employer		Relationship to Patient
		Father

INSURANCE INFORMATION

Primary Insurance Carrier	Phone Number
Health First	1-800-123-7777

Address	City	State	Zip
1234 Insurance Boulevard	Anytown	AL	12345-1234

Policy Holder Name (if different from patient)	Phone	Date of Birth	Sex
James Brown	123-251-9686	10/5/1975	M

Policy Number	Group Number
NW9908272	16096T

Secondary Insurance Carrier	Phone Number

Address	City	State	Zip

Policy Holder Name (if different from patient)	Phone	Date of Birth	Sex

Policy Number	Group Number

I hereby give lifetime authorization for payment of insurance benefits to be made directly to Walden-Martin Medical Group, and any assisting physicians, for services rendered. I understand that I am financially responsible for all charges whether or not they are covered by insurance. In the event of default, I agree to pay all costs of collection, and reasonable attorney's fees. I hereby authorize this healthcare provider to release all information necessary to secure the payment of benefits. I further agree that a photocopy of this agreement shall be as valid as the original.

Signature	Date
Christina Brown	

HealthFirst

MEMBER NAME: Brown, James
POLICY NUMBER: NW9908272
GROUP #: 16096T
DEPENDENTS: Brown, Christina   **EFFECTIVE DATE:** 11/24/2021

Network Coinsurance: DRUG CO-PAY
In: 80% / 20%   GENERIC: $20
Out: 60% / 40%   NAME BRAND: $50

CLAIMS/INQUIRIES: 1-800-123-7777

Figure 1.5 Patient information form and insurance card for Christina Brown.

The Browns have arrived for Christina's appointment and James has completed the Patient Information Form (Fig. 1.5). You will need to enter the demographic information into the electronic health record.

Checking in Christina Brown

1. Click the **Patient Demographics** icon.
2. Enter "Brown" in the **Last Name** field and click the **Search Existing Patients** button.
3. Christina's name should appear in blue. Click on **Christina**. There are three tabs for patient demographic information: **Patient, Guarantor,** and **Insurance**. All three have mandatory fields. Complete all of the mandatory fields (*) on the **Patient** tab and enter any other information that is supplied on the Patient Information Form.
4. Click on the **Guarantor** tab, complete all mandatory fields, and enter any other information that is supplied on the Patient Information Form. Because Christina is a minor, she is not responsible for her medical bills. James Brown is the guarantor. For the **Relationship of Guarantor to Patient**, the **Parent** radio button should be selected.
5. For the **Guarantor/Account #**, the **Create a new Guarantor** radio button should be selected.
6. Using the **Responsible Party Information** on the Patient Information form, complete the guarantor information required fields.
7. Complete the **Provider Information** section.
8. Click on the **Insurance** tab, complete all mandatory fields, and enter any other information that is supplied on the Patient Information Form.
9. Click on the **Save Patient** button. You will see a confirmation message. Click the **Yes** button.

Task 1.10 Reschedule an Appointment

Mr. Brown calls back later in the day to say that a meeting has just been scheduled for the Wednesday on which Christina's appointment is scheduled. He would like to reschedule the appointment for the following week.

Using the process you learned in Task 1.2, reschedule Christina Brown's appointment to following Wednesday.

You have had a busy first day on your practicum! You now have a firm handle on how the scheduling system works for setting up the appointment matrix, scheduling established and new patients, rescheduling patients, and registering new patients. Congratulations!

2. Day Two

Task 2.1 Scheduling New Patient Appointments and Generating Appropriate Forms

Today you will continue to work with the schedule. Jill would like you to learn about how the electronic health record (EHR) can be used to create forms and letters. Your first task is to schedule an appointment for a new patient and generate the forms needed for that patient.

The first call you take today is from Jon Wilson, who would like to schedule an annual examination with Dr. Martin. Jon is a new patient of the Walden-Martin Family Medical Clinic and has provided you with the following information:

Date of birth: 08/01/1986
Address:
987 Country Lane
Anytown, AL 12345-1234
Phone: 123-424-3098
Email: jwilson@wirefox.mail
Emergency contact: Elizabeth Wilson
Emergency contact phone: 123-424-3078
Language: English
Race: White
Ethnicity: Not Hispanic or Latino
Employer: Anytown Technical College
Insurance:
MetLife
1234 Insurance Avenue
Anytown, AL 12345
Phone: 800-123-4444
Policyholder: Jon Wilson
Social Security number: 555-87-4298
Policy/ID number: SP12458679
Group number: 487956

Jon would like to have an appointment on a Wednesday, as this is his day off from work. Access Dr. Martin's schedule and find an available time for this appointment next Wednesday. Remember that a new patient visit as well as an annual examination will take 45 minutes.

Both New Patient Visit and Annual Exam are possible appointment types. In this situation, New Patient Visit would provide a better description.

Schedule a New Patient Appointment

1. Open Dr. Martin's schedule.
2. Find the first available 45-minute appointment for today and click on that time slot.
3. Enter the information necessary to schedule an appointment for this patient. The appointment will appear on the calendar (refer to Task 1.6).

Before moving on to the next step you will need to complete the demographic information for Jon Wilson. Using the information provided above, click the **Patient Demographics** icon (Fig. 2.1), perform a patient search, select the patient name displayed in blue, and complete the three tabs in the Patient Demographics window (refer to Task 1.7).

Generate Appropriate Forms

As Jon is a new patient of the clinic and has an appointment scheduled in the future, Jill informs you that several forms should be sent to Jon prior to his appointment. The Walden-Martin Family Medical Clinic sends all new patients a New Patient Welcome letter, the Notice of Privacy Practices, a Patient Bill of Rights, and a Medical Records Release form. Your next task is to prepare these documents to send to Jon Wilson.

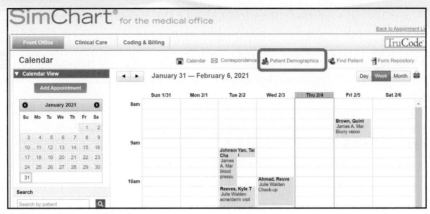

Figure 2.1 Patient Demograhics icon.

New Patient Welcome Letter. The New Patient Welcome letter tells the new patient what documents they need to bring with them to the appointment and gives them some general information about Walden-Martin Family Medical Clinic.

1. Click on the **Correspondence** icon, click on **Letters**, and then click on **New Patient Welcome**.
2. Perform a **Patient Search** for Jon Wilson, verify the autopopulated information, and add any missing information.
3. Click the **Save to Patient Record** button.

You have successfully used the EHR to create a letter.

Notice of Privacy Practices. It is a Health Insurance Portability and Accountability Act (HIPAA) requirement that all patients receive the clinic's Notice of Privacy Practices. The Walden-Martin Family Medical Clinic chooses to send this to new patients prior to their appointment. You will prepare this notice to be included with the Welcome letter.

1. Click on the **Form Repository** icon, then click on **Notice of Privacy Practice**.
2. Perform a **Patient Search** for Jon Wilson.
3. Click the **Save to Patient Record** button.

Patient Bill of Rights. The Walden-Martin Family Medical Clinic also sends new patients the Patient Bill of Rights document.

1. Locate the **Patient Bill of Rights** form and perform a **Patient Search**.
2. Click the **Save to Patient Record** button.

Medical Records Release. It is also the policy at the Walden-Martin Family Medical Clinic to send new patients a Medical Records Release form so that any previous medical records can be sent to the clinic.

1. Locate the **Medical Records Release** form and perform a **Patient Search**.
2. Confirm the autopopulated information and complete the form for all of Jon's previous records.
3. Click the **Save to Patient Record** button.

To view the documents you have just created, click on the **Find Patient** icon and do a **Patient Search** for Jon Wilson. You will land on the Patient Dashboard of the EHR. By scrolling down the page, you will see the New Patient Welcome letter in the Correspondence section and the three forms you created in the Forms section. You can click on any of them to print them out if required by your instructor (Fig. 2.2).

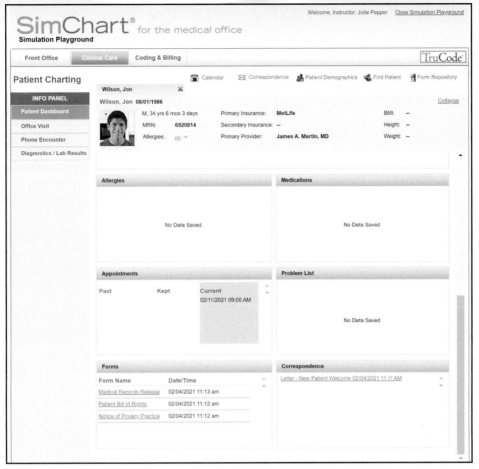

Figure 2.2 New Patient Welcom letter documentation in the Correspondence section.

Task 2.2 Creating Reminder Letters

Now that you are familiar with using letter templates, Jill would like you to create letters to remind patients of their upcoming appointments. You will be creating Appointment Reminder letters for the following patients:

- Quinton Brown
- Casey Hernandez
- Jana Green
1. Locate the Appointment Reminder letter template in Correspondence.
2. Perform a Patient Search for Quinton Brown.
3. Click on the next upcoming appointment from the Select Appointments—Scheduled list.
4. Click the Save to Patient Record button.
   Repeat this task for Casey Hernandez and Jana Green.

Scheduling Urgent Appointments

Sometimes a patient needs to be seen on the same day, as soon as possible. Box 2.1 gives some examples of conditions that should be seen on the same day.

BOX 2.1

Same-Day Appointments

- Sprains and strains
- Wounds without fracture or dislocation
- Nausea, vomiting, or diarrhea that has persisted for more than 2 or 3 days
- Fever
- Sudden illness or severe pain without bleeding, fainting, or loss of consciousness
- Sore throat, especially with fever
- Burning, frequency, or urgency associated with urination, especially if accompanied by fever or blood in the urine
- Vaginal bleeding in a pregnant woman

Amma Patel, DOB 01/14/1996, has called in stating that she is 22 weeks pregnant and noticed some vaginal bleeding and cramping this morning. Dr. Walden is her physician. This type of situation usually warrants double-booking the physician. Double-booking happens when two patients are scheduled at the same time for the same physician.

1. Schedule Amma Patel for an Urgent Visit as soon as possible today with Dr. Walden, even if it means double-booking. Remember that the Chief Complaint is the reason that the patient is being seen (refer to Task 1.3).

Task 2.4 Scheduling an Urgent Appointment for a Sick Patient

Maria Gomez has called in stating that her son Pedro, DOB 07/01/2016, has had a sore throat and temperature of 101.2 °F for 2 days. Walden-Martin Family Medical Clinic's policy states that those symptoms require a same-day appointment. Pedro usually sees Dr. Martin.

1. Schedule Pedro Gomez for an Urgent Visit as soon as possible with Dr. Martin. Maria has requested early afternoon so she can arrange for someone to watch her other children.

 PROFESSIONALISM

When dealing with an upset patient on the telephone, it is important for you to remain calm and collected. You should show the appropriate concern for the patient without upsetting the patient further. Empathy is important when dealing with a patient who is in a stressful situation.

Scheduling appointments is one of the activities that is often done when you are responsible for answering the telephones in a medical office. Another is updating the patient's demographic information when there has been a change in address, employer, insurance, and so on. Jill feels that you are ready to take on this task. You will be using many of the skills you have already learned. You will need to locate established patients and then update the demographic information that has changed.

Update the following patient demographic information:

> Monique Jones
> Date of birth: 06/23/1993
> Employer: Anytown Attorneys
> Primary insurance:
> Aetna
> 1234 Insurance Way
> Anytown, AL 12345
> Phone: 800-123-2222
> Policy/ID number: 4258796
> Group number: JK71133

1. Click on the **Patient Demographics** icon and search for Monique Jones, then click on the patient name displayed in blue to update and edit the demographics.
2. After all three sections are complete and updated, click the **Save Patient** button.

Update the following patient demographic information:

> Diego Lupez
> Date of birth: 08/01/1991
> Address:
> 482 Grant Avenue
> Anytown, AL 12345
> Home phone: 123-838-0449

1. Using the information above, update the **Patient Demographics**.
2. After the information is updated, click the **Save Patient** button.

Locate the **Telephone Messages** area on the companion Evolve website (Task 2.6). These are the nonurgent messages that came into the clinic during the hours in which the clinic was closed. Jill has asked you to listen to the messages and complete a Phone Message for each in the EHR.

1. Click on the **Correspondence** icon to locate **Phone Messages** in the information panel on the left side of the screen and perform a **Patient Search**.
2. Document the information accurately.
3. If a patient requests a specific time for an appointment, schedule the appointment as close as possible to the time requested by the patient. Indicate the date and time of the appointment in the **Action Documentation** section of the **Phone Message**.
4. Click the **Save to Patient Record** button.

You have done a great job documenting the phone messages. Jill has asked you to now go back to answering live calls. Your first call is from Sofia Hernandez. Her daughter Casey Hernandez, DOB 10/08/2009, was treated by Jean Burke, NP, for influenza. Casey was initially seen 1 week ago and is now able to return to school on Monday of next week with no restrictions. Casey's school is asking for a Certificate to Return to School, so they have documentation that the provider feels that Casey is ready to return to school.

1. Click on the **Forms Repository** icon and locate the **Certificate to Return to Work or School** template.
2. Click on the **Patient Search** button at the bottom of the form and search for Casey Hernandez, DOB 10/08/2009.
3. Complete the open fields with the information provided above.
4. Click the **Save to Patient Record** button.

The next call you receive is from Walter Biller, DOB 01/04/1978. He will be moving out of town in a few weeks and would like to get his medical records transferred to his new provider. Use the information below to complete the Medical Records Release form to send to Mr. Biller for his signature so you can then send his records to his new provider. Remember that you are releasing the records from Walden-Martin Family Medical Clinic to the new provider.

New Provider:
Chippewa Valley Family Medicine Clinic
619 Clinic Avenue
Eau Claire, WI 54701-1234
Phone: 555-987-6759
Fax: 555-987-4568
Expiration date: One year from today

1. Locate the **Medical Records Release** form and perform a **Patient Search**.
2. Confirm the autopopulated information and complete the form for all of Mr. Biller's records from Walden-Martin Family Medical Clinic.
3. Click the **Save to Patient Record** button.

You have handled all the tasks that have been given to you very well! Jill would like to introduce you to another role that has become an integral part of the healthcare team. The addition of medical scribes to the healthcare team has allowed providers to focus more closely on the patient. Many patients feel that providers are spending more time interacting with the computer than with them. This has led to the development of the medical scribe profession.

A scribe's responsibilities could include the following:
- Assisting the provider in navigating the EHR
- Entering information into the EHR as directed by the provider
  - History of the present illness
  - Review of systems
  - Vital signs
  - Lab results
  - Diagnostic imaging results
  - Progress notes
  - Care plans
  - Medication lists
- Locating information within the EHR for provider review (laboratory and test results)
- Responding to patient requests for information as directed by the provider

A medical scribe should have an understanding of medical terminology, excellent computer skills, and strong attention to detail. It is important for medical scribes to understand that they are not obtaining the information from the patient. Their role is to document the information from the provider and enter the information into the EHR, per the provider's instructions.

Healthcare facilities that have hired scribes have found that both the patients and providers are more satisfied with patient encounters. These providers can establish better relationships with patients because they are able to spend their time in face-to-face interaction rather than interacting with the computer.

At Walden-Martin Family Medical Clinic, those working in the administrative areas are sometimes asked to fill in as scribes. Jill would like you to work with Dr. Kahn as his medical scribe.

For this task, you will be using the Clinical Care tab in SimChart for the Medical Office (Fig. 2.3).

You have documented the chief complaint previously when you have scheduled appointments. That information is used to determine how much time should be allotted for the appointment. After the patient has arrived and is meeting with their provider, the chief complaint is reassessed and documented in the Clinical Care section of the EHR. Along with the chief complaint, the provider will explore the history of the present illness. This is the chronological description of the patient's present illness from the first symptoms to the present. There are several components to the history of the present illness:

- Location
- Quality
- Severity
- Duration
- Timing
- Context
- Modifying factors
- Associated signs and symptoms

The provider will also be doing a review of systems. This is basically an inventory of the body systems that is assessed with a series of questions to identify signs and/or symptoms that the patient may be experiencing.

For this task, you will be working as a scribe to document the information about the chief complaint, history of present illness, and review of systems that provider gains while talking with the patient.

1. Click on the **Clinical Care** tab and locate Celia Tapia's name in the List of Patients. Click on the radio button next to her name and then click on the **Select** button.
2. In order to enter the information into the EHR, you will need to create an encounter. Click on **Office Visit** in the Info Panel.
3. Select **Follow-up/Established Visit** for the Visit Type and **David Kahn, MD** for the Provider, and click on the **Save** button. At this time, the medical record will open up and the Record drop-down menu will appear.
4. Click on **Chief Complaint** from the Record drop-down menu.
5. Click in the textbox under **Chief Complaint**. Celia tells Dr. Kahn that she decided to come in and see him today because she has been having a sore throat, cough, fever with chills, fatigue, and body aches for the past 3 days and isn't getting better. Dr. Kahn asks you to document that in the Chief Complaint section. Remember to use quotation marks around statements that are in the patient's own words.
6. Dr. Kahn then moves on to the **History of the Present Illness**. He asks her about her symptoms. The body aches are all over her body and she describes them as muscle aches. Click in the **Location** section of the History of Present Illness to document this information.

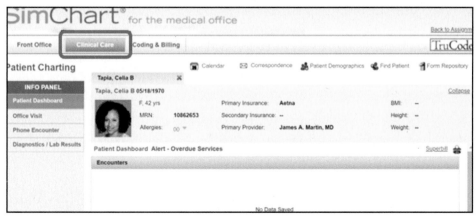

Figure 2.3 Clinical Care tab.

7. Click in the **Quality** section to document that the patient describes the pain as an ache.
8. Click on the **Severity** section to document that the patient describes it as a 3 on a scale of 1–10.
9. Click on the **Duration** section to document 3 days.
10. Click on the **Associated Signs and Symptoms** section to document the fever, chills, and cough.
11. To document the Review of Systems information, you will be clicking on the radio button next to sign/symptoms. Click **Yes** to indicate that the patient has that sign/symptom and **No** to indicate that they do not. Dr. Kahn asks you to click Yes to the following: in the General section—fever, chills, fatigue; in the HEENT (head, eyes, ears, nose, and throat) section—sore throat; in the Resp (respiratory) section—cough; and in the MS (musculoskeletal system)—myalgia (muscle aches and pain). The **No** radio button can be clicked for all of the others.
12. Click the **Save** button.

You have successfully documented the chief complaint, history of present illness, and review of systems as a scribe! Dr. Kahn thanks you for helping him with this patient.

Based on Celia's signs/symptoms, Dr. Kahn has ordered a rapid strep test and it has come back positive for strep throat. He has ordered a prescription for amoxicillin (Augmentin) 500 mg by mouth every 12 hours for 10 days. He has asked you, as the scribe, to update the medication list to show this new medication.

1. Click on the **Record** drop-down menu and select **Medications** from the list. Make sure that you are in the **Prescription Medication** tab.
2. Click on the **Add Medication** button.
3. In the **Add Prescription Medication** window, search for amoxicillin in the **Medication** field. Select **Amoxicillin/Clavulanate potassium Tablet—(Augmentin)** from the drop-down menu.
4. Select **500** from the drop-down menu for **Strength**.
5. Select **Tablet** from the drop-down menu for **Form**.
6. Select **Oral** from the drop-down menu for **Route**.
7. Select **Every 12 Hours** from the drop-down menu for **Frequency**.
8. Enter **500 mg by mouth every 12 hours** in the **Dose** field.
9. Select today's date from the Calendar picker in the **Start Date** field.
10. Enter **Strep Throat** in the **Indication** field.
11. Click on the **Active** radio button in the **Status** section.
12. Click on the **Save** button.

You have successfully documented the chief complaint, history of present illness, and review of systems, as well as updated the medication list as a scribe! Dr. Kahn thanks you for helping him with this patient.

You have learned some new aspects of the EHR today, and you will be able to apply those skills in the coming days. Well done!

3. Day Three

Risk Management

Today, Jill wants you to develop a better understanding of risk management in the medical office. You remember discussing risk management in school, but Jill would like you to see how those principles are applied in the actual clinic.

Risk is anything that may result in injury, illness, or financial loss to the clinic. Risk management involves policies and procedures that are in place to reduce those risks. You already followed some of the risk management policies when you prepared the appropriate forms for the new patient Jon Wilson by including the Notice of Privacy Practices and Medical Records Release forms with his New Patient Welcome letter. The Notice of Privacy Practices is required by HIPAA, and you are protecting the practice from a potential fine by documenting that the patient received it. By using the Medical Records Release form, you are protecting the office from an accusation of breach of confidentiality.

There are several other forms that are used in risk management, such as the Disclosure Authorization and the Incident Report.

Task 3.1 Disclosure Authorization

A Disclosure Authorization form should be signed if a patient wants someone else, such as a family member, to have access to the medical records, or to allow health professionals to discuss the patient's condition with someone other than the patient.

Quinton Brown, DOB 02/24/1986, is an established patient of Dr. Martin. Quinton has had some recent health issues and would like his partner, Jon Angleston, to be able to have access to his records and discuss any issues with Dr. Martin. A Disclosure Authorization form will need to be completed.

> Jon Angleston
> Address:
> 4554 Browning Street
> Anytown, AL 12345

1. Find the **Disclosure Authorization** in the **Form Repository** and perform a **Patient Search**.
2. Review the autopopulated fields and complete all other required fields.
3. Click the **Save to Patient Record** button.

The Disclosure Authorization has now been saved to Quinton Brown's record and can be used to give information to Jon Angleston when he requests it.

After Amma Patel's pregnancy scare, she decided that she would like her husband to be able speak to the doctor about her pregnancy. Complete the Disclosure Authorization form.

> Gopal Patel
> Address:
> 1346 Charity Lane
> Anytown, AL 12345

1. Find the **Disclosure Authorization** in the **Form Repository** and perform a **Patient Search**.
2. Review the autopopulated fields and complete all other required fields.
3. Click the **Save to Patient Record** button.

Task 3.2 Incident Report

An Incident Report is a document that is used to report any issues that affect patient or staff safety within the clinic. It provides documentation of what happened and can be used to develop safety measures so that the same problem does not occur again. The Incident Report form can be found in the Office Forms section of the Form Repository.

While you are sitting at the front desk, you witness a patient slip and fall as he enters the clinic. It is a rainy day, and the entryway floor is quite wet. Use the following information to complete the Incident Report:

Today's date and time:
Department: Family practice
Medical team: Dr. Martin
Patient reason for visit: Appointment
Immediate actions: Dr. Martin assessed patient injuries. Minor bruising found. No additional treatment needed.
Contributing factors: Water in the entryway.
Prevention: Mats in entryway to absorb water.
Next of kin/guardian notified/patient: No
Medical staff notified: Yes
Contact phone number: 123-123-1234
Other persons involved: None
Position: N/A
Medical report: Minor bruising, no treatment.
Designation: Accidental
Check the Signature on File box

---

1. Find the **Incident Form** in the **Form Repository**.
2. Complete all required fields. It is important to be specific and detailed in the documentation of an Incident Report.
3. Click the **Save** button.

An Incident Report is not part of the patient's medical record, so it is saved to a central location within the office, rather than the patient record. In SimChart for the Medical Office, reference past incident reports by clicking the Saved Forms tab (Fig. 3.1). Although it is not part of the patient record, it is still very important to document the incident accurately and objectively. The Incident Report is saved to be used as a tool to prevent the occurrence from happening again. It may be used to develop new policies and procedures to protect both patients and staff.

Referral Forms

Another form that is often needed is a referral form. This form is used when one provider wants a patient to see another provider. It is often required by insurance carriers, especially managed care organizations, before they agree to pay for services from the new provider.

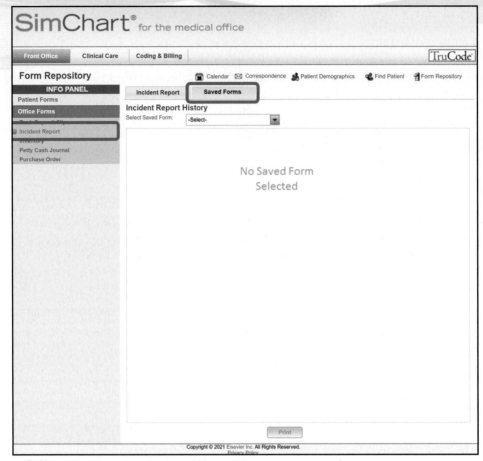

Figure 3.1 Incident Reports in the Saved Forms tab.

Task 3.3 Referral Form

Dr. Walden would like her patient Carl Bowden, DOB 04/05/1963, to see an endocrinologist for issues related to his type 2 diabetes. The endocrinologist is Dr. Casper at Anytown Endocrinology Clinic, 3661 Grant Avenue, Anytown, AL 12345. She would like to refer Carl for 10 visits.

> Diagnosis: Type 2 diabetes, uncontrolled; ICD-9 250.02, ICD-10 E11.65
> Significant clinical information/symptoms: Uncontrolled blood glucose levels, Hgb A1c 11.2%
> Medications: Glimepiride 2 mg daily
> Walden-Martin Family Medical Clinic, Phone 123-123-1234
> Dr. Walden's NPI number: 987654321

1. Find the **Referral** form in the **Form Repository** and perform a **Patient Search**.
2. Using the information provided above, complete all necessary fields.
3. Click the **Save to Patient Record** button.

Written Communication

When working in a healthcare facility, you are often required to use written communication. This could be a letter or an email to patients, other providers, coworkers, or supply companies. Many EHR systems, including SimChart, use templates for the most common types of communication. These templates are found by clicking on the Correspondence icon (Fig. 3.2). This keeps the messages clear and uniform. Tasks 3.4 and 3.5 will get you familiar with using the template format for written communication.

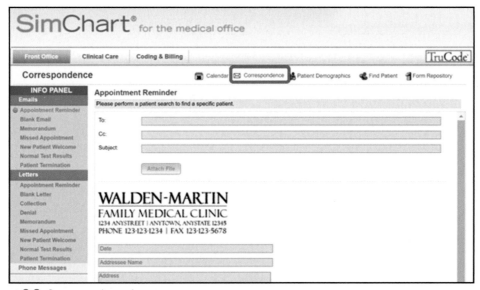

Figure 3.2 Correspondence icon.

Task 3.4 Missed Appointment Letter

Mora Siever missed her 3:30 PM appointment with Jean Burke, NP, yesterday afternoon. It is Walden-Martin Family Medical Clinic's policy to send a letter to patients who have missed an appointment. This serves two purposes: it documents the fact that the patient did not show up for a scheduled appointment and gives the patient the opportunity to reschedule the appointment. Jill would like you to generate a Missed Appointment letter for Mora.

1. Find the **Missed Appointment** letter in **Correspondence** and perform a **Patient Search**.
2. Complete all necessary fields.
3. Click the **Save to Patient Record** button.

Task 3.5 Memorandum Email

The providers at Walden-Martin Family Medical Clinic want to show their appreciation to all of the staff by hosting a picnic for all employees and their families. The picnic will be held 2 weeks from this coming Saturday from 11:00 AM until 4:00 PM at the Anytown Park. There will be burgers and hot dogs cooked on the grill, chips, salads, fruit, and beverages provided. There will also be games for both the adults and children. The providers hope that everyone will be able to come and enjoy some down time with their coworkers. The clinic will be closed for that Saturday so that all can participate. They would like to get RSVPs by the Thursday before the picnic so that they know how much food to prepare.

Jill has asked you to prepare an email memorandum to be sent to all of the staff telling them about the picnic and asking for the RSVP. Staff can just reply to the email with their response. Use the Email Memorandum template and compose the email to be sent to everyone. Remember that grammar and punctuation are very important with all forms of written communication.

1. Locate the **Email Memorandum** template in **Correspondence**.
2. Complete all of the fields and compose a professional message containing all of the information about the picnic.
3. Click on the **Save** button.

Coding and Billing Responsibilities

Another important administrative function is completing the Superbill and Ledger to document the services provided for billing purposes. The provider may complete the Superbill or it may be the office staff's job to complete. The information from the Superbill is then posted to the account ledger, where a running total of the charges for the services provided and payments made on the account are recorded. After the charges have been recorded in the superbill and on the ledger, a claim needs to be created so that the insurance company can be billed. The following exercises will walk you through that process.

Task 3.6 Preparing a Superbill

Truong Tran (DOB 05/30/2000) was seen today by Dr. Kahn for an ingrown toenail. As this is a fairly straightforward visit Jill has asked you to complete the Superbill for this visit. Using the information below complete the Superbill to show the services provided and amount charged for each. Before you can complete the Superbill, you will need to create an encounter in the Clinical Care module (see Task 2.9), before moving to the Coding and Billing module (Fig. 3.3).

Diagnoses: Ingrowing nail L60.0
Office Visit: 99212 $32.00
Copay: $10.00
Same Name as Patient
Same Address as Patient

---

1. Click on the **Clinical Care** module and perform a search to locate Truong Tran (DOB 5/30/2000). Click on the radio button next to his name and then click on the **Select** button.
2. To create an encounter, click on **Office Visit** in the Info Panel. If encounters already exist for Truong you will need to click on the **Add New** tab.
3. Select **Follow-up/Established Visit** for the Visit Type and **David Kahn, MD** for the Provider and click on the Save button.
4. After the encounter has been created click on the **Coding and Billing** module (Figure 3-3) and locate Truong Tran.
5. From the list of **Encounters Not Coded** click on the one you created today. This will open up the Superbill.
6. On page 1 of the Superbill you will be entering the diagnosis by clicking on the ICD-10 radio button and then entering **Ingrowing nail L60.0**.
7. In the **Office Visit** section enter a **Rank** of **1** next to Problem focused, the fee of **$32.00** and the procedure code of **99212** in the Est column. Click **Save**.
8. Click **Next** three times to get to page 4.
9. Enter the **$10.00** in the **Copay** field.
10. Enter **0.00** in the **Previous Balance** field and **32.00** in the **Balance Due** field.
11. In the next section click, in the **Same Name as Patient** box and in the **Same Address as Patient** box.
12. In the next section click on the radio button for **Self** in the **Patient Relationship to Insured** area. Click in the **Married** box in the **Patient Status** area. Click the **No** radio button in the **Is there another health benefit plan?** area.
13. Enter **123-456-1237** in the Telephone section.
14. In the next section click the **No** radio button for **Employment?, Auto Accident?,** and **Other Accident?**
15. Click in the **I am ready to submit the Superbill** box, then click the **Yes** radio button in the **Signature on file:** section and use today's date in the **Date:** section.
16. Click the **Save** button and then click on the **Submit Superbill** button.

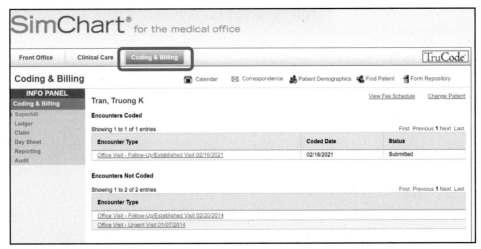

Figure 3.3 Coding and Billing module.

Truong paid his $10.00 copayment while he was at the office. This needs to be posted to his ledger.

1. While in the Coding and Billing module, click on **Ledger** in the Info Panel.
2. Perform a **Patient Search** to locate Truong's ledger. Click on the radio button next to his name and then click on the **Select** button.
3. To open the ledger, click on the arrow to the right of Truong Tran's name. This will open up the ledger.
4. Click in the gray box under **Transaction Date** to open the calendar picker and choose today's date.
5. Click in the gray box under **DOS** (date of service) to open the calendar picker and choose today's date.
6. Select **David Kahn, MD** from the Provider drop-down menu.
7. Select **PTPYMTCK** from the Service drop-down menu.
8. Enter **10.00** in the Payment column.
9. Click the **Save** button.

Now that the Superbill has been completed and the copayment posted to the ledger, it is time to prepare the insurance claim for Truong Tran's services.

1. Select **Claim** from the information panel on the left side of the screen and perform a **Patient Search** for Truong Tran. You will see the encounter for today with the status of **Not Started**. Click on the paper and pencil icon to open the claim.
2. The claim consists of seven tabs. Review the autopopulated information for the Patient Info, Provider Info, Payer Info, Encounter Notes, and Claim Info tabs. Add any missing information and click the **Save** button for each tab.
3. On the **Charge Capture** tab, enter today's date as the DOS From and DOS To.
4. Enter **99212** in the **CPT/HCPCS** column.
5. Click the **Place of Service** link to determine the correct the POS (place of service) code. Enter the correct code in the POS column.
6. Enter **1** in the DX column. This refers to ranking of the diagnosis found on the Encounter Notes page.
7. Enter **32.00** in the Fee column.
8. Enter **1** in the Units column.
9. Click the **Save** button.
10. Click on the **Submission** tab and click the checkbox next to **I am ready to submit the Claim**.
11. Select the **Yes** radio button in the Signature on File field and enter today's date in the Date field.
12. Click the **Submit Claim** button.

Task 3.9 Preparing the Superbill for Missed Charges

Jill has been auditing patient accounts to make sure that all patient visits have been billed, and she has found a visit on 01/09/2022 for Dr. Martin's patient Amma Patel, DOB 01/14/1996, that has no Superbill or Ledger entries. She was seen for iron deficiency anemia and she did not make a payment that day. The Superbill can be found by clicking on the Coding and Billing module (Fig. 3.3).

Previous balance: 0.00
Services provided:
Established patient, problem-focused office visit - 99212
Insurance:
Blue Cross Blue Shield
1234 Insurance Place
Anytown, AL 12345
Phone: 800-123-1111
Amma is the insured, ID number is WMF456987123, Group number is MW55874.
Condition is not related to employment, auto accident, or other accident.
Diagnosis: Iron deficiency anemia; ICD-10 D50.9
HIPAA form is on file, date 01/09/2022

---

1. Click on the **Coding and Billing** module, then **Superbill** from the Info Panel on the left side of the screen, and do a **Patient Search**.
2. Under the **Encounters Not Coded** grid, click on **Comprehensive Visit—Follow-up/Established Visit 01/09/2022**. This will open up the Superbill.
3. Complete the Superbill following the same process as used for Truong Tran.

Task 3.10 Preparing an Insurance Claim for Missed Charges

Because a Superbill was never created, an insurance claim was not sent either. The next step would be to prepare the insurance claim. You will be using information from the Superbill and from the box below to complete the insurance claim process.

Billing Provider Information:
Julie Walden
Walden-Martin Family Medical Clinic
1234 Anystreet
Anytown, AL 12345-1234
Phone: 123-123-1234

1. Select **Claim** from the information panel on the left side of the screen and perform a **Patient Search**. You will see the encounter for DOS 01/09/2022 with the status of Not Started. Click on the paper and pencil icon to open the claim.
2. Review the autopopulated information for the Patient Info, Provider Info, Payer Info, Encounter Notes, and Claim Info tabs. Add any missing information and click the **Save** button for each tab.
3. Complete the **Charge Capture** tab, using the same process as Truong Tran.
4. Click on the **Submission** tab and click the checkbox next to **I am ready to submit the Claim**.
5. Select the **Yes** radio button in the Signature on File field and enter **01/09/2022** in the Date field.
6. Click the **Submit Claim** button.

   This has been another information-packed day! You have learned about risk management and have been introduced to the electronic billing process. Good work!

4. Day Four

There are many different ways of communicating information to patients. It can be done with a phone call, a traditional letter, messaging through the patient portal, or an email. The use of email and patient portal messages to communicate with patients is on the rise in healthcare. In the past, email had not been considered confidential, and maintaining patient confidentiality is key in healthcare. However, more and more patients want to receive information quickly and in the format with which they are most comfortable, and for many that is email. In addition, as part of the Health Information Technology for Economic and Clinical Health (HITECH) Act and Meaningful Use, eligible professionals are required to use secure electronic messaging to communicate with patients regarding relevant health information. This could be email or through the patient portal. A patient portal is a secure website where a patient can access personal health information, schedule appointments, refill prescriptions 24 hours a day, and message their healthcare providers. Oftentimes it is part of the provider's electronic health record.

Jill explains to you that it is the policy of the Walden-Martin Family Medical Clinic to relay information to patients using the secure email system within the electronic health record if the patient has given permission to do so. The patient must also supply the clinic with the proper email address to use. The patient will sign a form giving permission for emails to be sent to a specific email address. The patient can choose to use email for appointment reminders, normal laboratory test results, and answers to questions.

When Jon Wilson was in for his annual examination, Dr. Martin ordered a lipid profile based on Jon's family history of coronary artery disease. The results have come back from the outside laboratory and all are normal. Jon has given permission for his test results to be emailed to him and he would like a copy of the results sent as well. Jill asks that you send out the email with the results as an attachment.

Sending an Email with an Attachment

The electronic health record has several templates already set up for the most common types of emails and letters that the clinic sends out. The normal test results template is one of these types.

1. Find the **Normal Test Results** template by clicking on the **Correspondence** icon (Fig. 4.1), locating the template, and performing a **Patient Search**.
2. Review the autopopulated fields and complete all other required fields.
3. Click on the **Attach File** button, then click on the **Browse** button and locate the laboratory results file (found on the Evolve website, Task 4.1; you must save this document to your computer or storage device before attaching it to this email). Click on the **Upload** button.
4. Click the **Send** button and a copy of the email will be saved to the patient record.

Some patients will still want to be contacted using the regular mail system. Templates can be used for this as well. You would need to print out the letter and an envelope, and put it in the mail. If the letter is created using the EHR system, a copy will automatically be saved to the patient's record. If the letter is created outside of the EHR system, it would have to be scanned in and then uploaded to the patient's record.

Jill has asked that you send a letter to a patient regarding her normal test results. While there is a template for a normal test results letter, Jill would like you to practice your professional letter-writing skills by using the Blank Letter template. The letter should go to Julia Berkley (DOB 07/05/1998), who recently had thyroid function tests done, all of which were normal.

1. Find the **Blank Letter** template by clicking on the **Correspondence** icon (Fig. 4.1), locating the template under the **Letters** heading, and performing a **Patient Search**.
2. Review the autopopulated fields.
3. Compose a professional letter informing Ms. Berkley that her recent thyroid function tests were all normal and if she has any questions, she should contact Dr. Martin.
4. Proofread your letter and when you are satisfied, click on **Save to Patient Record** button.
5. Click on **OK** button when the **Date Selection** pop-up window opens up.
6. To print the letter, click on the **Find Patient** button, perform a **Patient Search** for Julia Berkley, then scroll down to the **Correspondence** section of the Dashboard, click on the letter you just created, and then click on the **Print** button.

◎ PROFESSIONALISM

Email tips: Written communication is just as important as face-to-face communication. Maintaining a professional demeanor is harder to do when you do not have body language to help convey your message. It is important to proofread any written communication before it is sent out. If you are unsure if it conveys the message you really want, you should have someone else read it as well. If you are unsure about the spelling of any words, look them up in a dictionary. Do not completely rely on the software's spell-check, as it will not indicate if you are using the word correctly (e.g., there, their, or they're).

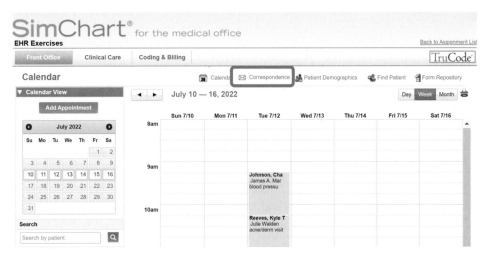

Figure 4.1 The correspondence icon.

Day Four

Locate the **Telephone Messages** area on the companion Evolve website (Task 4.3). These are the nonurgent messages the clinic received last evening. As this is a task you have done before, Jill would like you to listen to the messages, complete a Phone Message for each in the electronic health record, schedule the appointment, and respond to the patient.

1. Click on the **Correspondence** icon to locate **Phone Messages** on the left side of the screen (Fig. 4.2) and perform a **Patient Search**.
2. Document the information accurately.
3. Schedule the appointment as close as possible to the time requested by the patient. Indicate the date and time of the appointment in the **Action Documentation** section of the **Phone Message**.
4. Click the **Save to Patient Record** button.
5. Using the **Blank Email** template, compose a professional email indicating the date and time for which the appointment has been scheduled, which doctor it is scheduled with, and how the patient should contact the office to change the appointment if the time is inconvenient.
6. Click the **Send** button.
7. You can view the email by clicking on **Find Patient**, doing a **Patient Search**, and then scrolling down to the **Correspondence** section of the Patient Dashboard.
    Complete these steps for all messages remaining for this task.

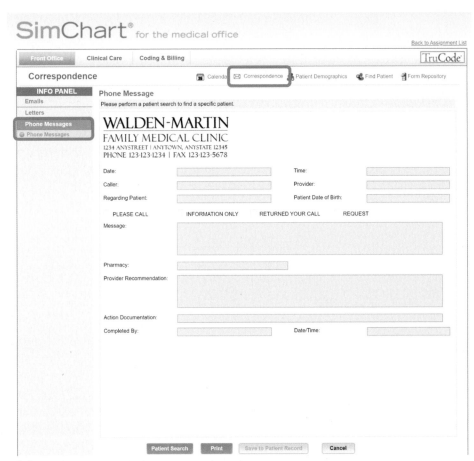

Figure 4.2 Phone messages in the correspondence icon.

After taking care of the phone messages, Jill wants you to answer the telephone requests for appointments. Your first call is from a new patient requesting an appointment with Dr. Walden for an annual examination.

Megan would like an appointment on any day at 11:00 AM. Access Dr. Walden's schedule and find an available day for this appointment. Remember that a new patient visit as well as an annual examination will take 45 minutes. Use the information below to schedule the appointment.

Patient name: Megan E. Adams
Date of birth: 09/27/1990
Address:
2310 Madison Avenue
Anytown, AL 12345
Phone: 123-435-5298
Emergency contact: Kevin Adams
Emergency contact phone: 123-435-6601
Employer: Anytown Hospital
Insurance:
Aetna
1234 Insurance Way
Anytown, AL 12345
Phone: 800-123-2222
Policy holder: Megan Adams
Social Security number: 444-92-5544
Policy/ID number: 0927198426
Group number: AH4218

Schedule a New Patient Appointment

1. Open Dr. Walden's schedule.
2. Find the first 45-minute appointment available at 11:00 AM. Click on that time slot.
3. Enter the information necessary to add this patient and appointment. The appointment will appear on the calendar (refer to Task 1.6).

As with the previous new patient, Jon Wilson, whom you scheduled, you will need to send Megan the appropriate forms. Before doing so, you will need to complete the demographic information for Megan Adams. Using the information provided, click on the **Patient Demographics** icon and complete the three tabs in this window (refer to Task 1.9).

Generate Appropriate Forms

Using the **Correspondence** and **Form Repository** icons, complete the New Patient Welcome letter, Notice of Privacy Practice form, Patient Bill of Rights, and the Medical Records Release form. Save all of the documents to Megan's record.

To view the documents you have just created, click on the **Find Patient** icon and perform a **Patient Search** for Megan Adams. You will land on the Patient Dashboard of the electronic health record. By scrolling down the page, you will see the New Patient Welcome letter in the Correspondence section and the three forms you created in the Forms section. You can click on any of them to print them out if required by your instructor.

Day Four

Schedule a New Patient Appointment and Generate Appropriate Forms

You take two more calls for new patients. Schedule the appointments using the information below.

Thomas would like an appointment on any day after 3:00 PM with Dr. Martin for a new patient visit to discuss his blood pressure. After the appointment has been scheduled, generate the appropriate forms for this new patient.

Patient name: Thomas R. Carter
Date of birth: 02/24/1957
Address:
221 9th Street W.
Anytown, AL 12345
Phone: 123-467-9731
Emergency contact: Donna Carter
Emergency contact phone: 123-435-3621
Employer: Anytown Middle School
Insurance:
Aetna
1234 Insurance Way
Anytown, AL 12345
Phone: 800-123-2222
Policy holder: Thomas Carter
Social Security number: 777-32-1597
Policy/ID number: 0224195146
Group number: MS2264

Peggy would like an appointment anytime on a Thursday with Jean Burke, NP, for a new patient visit. After the appointment has been scheduled, generate the appropriate forms for this new patient.

Patient name: Peggy Taylor
Date of birth: 01/12/1993
Address:
421 Main Street
Anytown, AL 12345
Phone: 123-552-1040
Social Security number: 989-22-8765
Emergency contact: Randy Taylor
Emergency contact phone: 123-552-6065
Employer: Anytown Accountants
Insurance:
Blue Cross Blue Shield
1234 Insurance Place
Anytown, AL 12345
Phone: 800-123-1111
Policy holder: Randy Taylor
Policy holder Social Security number: 898-44-6974
Policy/ID number: AAA587945
Group number: 45879FQ

Task 4.5 Documents Received in the Mail

With an electronic health record, many documents mailed to the clinic must be scanned and then uploaded to the medical record. Several documents have arrived in today's mail and have been scanned, and Jill would like you to upload them into the proper section of the patient's medical record.

Operative Report

During her last visit with Dr. Martin, Norma Washington, DOB 08/01/1953, mentioned that she had a hip replacement several years ago when she lived elsewhere. Dr. Martin wanted to see the operative report for that procedure and asked Norma to complete a Medical Records Release form. The operative report was received in the mail today and has been scanned. It now needs to be uploaded into the Health History section of Norma's record.

1. On the Evolve website, locate the documents for Task 4.5 and save them to your computer or storage device.
2. Click on the **Find Patient** icon and perform a **Patient Search**. The **Clinical Care** tab will open on the Patient Dashboard for Norma Washington.
3. To enter the health record, select the **Office Visit—Follow-up/Established Visit 01/22/2013** link within the **Encounters** section. The health record will open on the Allergies section displaying the **Record** drop-down menu (Fig. 4.3). Select **Health History** from the drop-down menu.
4. On the **Medical History** tab scroll down to **Past Surgeries** and click on the **Add New** button.
5. Enter the date of the surgery, found on the Operative Report, in the **Date** field. Enter "Left Hip Repair" in the **Type of Surgery** field.
6. Click on the **Browse** button in the **Upload Surgical Record** section. Locate the previously saved Operative Report and click the **Save** button.

Immunization Record

Also in today's mail is an immunization record for Casey Hernandez, DOB 10/08/2009. This has been scanned and now needs to be uploaded to Casey's record.

1. Click on the **Find Patient** icon and perform a **Patient Search**. The Clinical Care tab will open on the Patient Dashboard for Casey Hernandez.
2. Enter the health record by clicking on the **Encounter**. Select **Immunizations** from the **Record** drop-down menu and upload the immunization record that you had previously saved from the Evolve website.

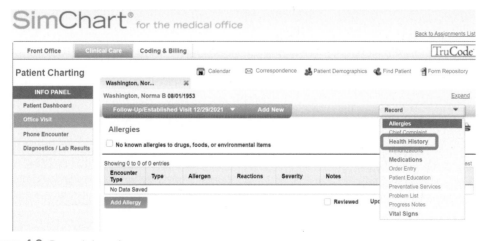

Figure 4.3 Record drop-down menu.

Laboratory Report

In preparation for his upcoming annual examination with Dr. Martin, Jon Wilson, DOB 08/01/1986, has had his previously performed lipid profile results sent to the Walden-Martin Family Medical Clinic. These results have been scanned and now need to be uploaded to his record.

1. Click on the **Find Patient** icon and perform a **Patient Search**. The **Clinical Care** tab will open on the Patient Dashboard for Jon Wilson.
2. Select **Diagnostics/Lab Results** from the information panel on the left side of the screen and click the **Add** button.
3. Enter the date of the lipid profile from the report in the **Date** field.
4. Select the appropriate **Type** from the drop-down menu and indicate "lipid profile" in the **Notes** field.
5. Upload the report that you had previously saved from the Evolve website and click the **Save** button.

When Al Neviaser, DOB 06/21/1976, was in the office 3 days ago, he mentioned to Dr. Martin that he was having some lower back pain. Dr. Martin told him that if it did not get better, he would order an MRI to see what was going on. Al has called to say that the pain is actually getting worse. Jill tells you that because it is documented in the medical record that Dr. Martin would like to order an MRI, you should proceed with completing the Prior Authorization form.

Many insurance companies require prior authorization for certain services, including inpatient hospitalizations, new or experimental procedures, and certain diagnostic studies. Al's insurance carrier requires prior authorization for an MRI.

1. Click on the **Form Repository** icon to locate the **Prior Authorization Request** and perform a **Patient Search**.
2. Use the information below to complete the form.

Ordering physician: James A. Martin
Provider contact name: Jill King
Place of service/treatment and address:
Anytown Hospital
2345 Anystreet
Anytown, AL 12345
Service requested: MRI of thoracic and lumbar spine
Diagnosis/ICD code: Lower back pain ICD-10 M54.5
Injury related?: No
Workers' Compensation related?: No

---

3. Click **Save to Patient Record**.

You have learned a number of new skills today! Jill is very pleased with how you have handled the tasks she gave you. For the rest of the day, Jill would like you to practice the skills that you have learned over the previous 3 days.

Reuven Ahmad, DOB 9/12/1976, is here today to be seen for a follow-up appointment. He had previously injured his foot while doing some home repairs and has not be able to work for the past 2 weeks. He is here today to see Julie Walden, MD, to find out when he can return to work and to get the documentation that his employer has requested indicating that he can safely return to work.

When Mr. Ahmad checks in for his appointment, he tells you that his address has changed since he was last at Walden-Martin. Using the information below, update Mr. Ahmad's address (refer to Task 2.5).

Reuven Ahmad
Address:
1942 Zera Lane
Anytown, AL 12345

Jill has asked that you act as a scribe for Mr. Ahmad's visit today. You will be documenting the chief complaint, history of present illness, and the review of systems for today's visit (refer to Task 2.9).

1. Click on the **Clinical Care** tab and locate Reuven Ahmad's name in the List of Patients. Click on the radio button next to his name and then click on the **Select** button.

2. In order to enter the information into the EHR, you will need to create an encounter. Click on **Office Visit** in the Info Panel.

3. Select **Follow-up/Established Visit** for the Visit Type and **Julie Walden, MD** for the Provider and click on the **Save** button. At this time, the medical record will open up and the Record drop-down menu will appear.

4. Click on **Chief Complaint** from the Record drop-down menu.

5. Click in the textbox under **Chief Complaint**. Reuven tells Dr. Walden that his left foot is feeling much better after dropping a heavy box on it 2 weeks ago, and he is able to stand on it for more than 2 hours at a stretch without pain. Dr. Walden asks you to document that in the Chief Complaint section. Remember to use quotation marks around statements that are in the patient's own words.

6. Dr. Walden then moves on to the **History of the Present Illness**. She asks him about his symptoms. Reuven states that the pain in his left foot is very minimal. Click in the **Location** section of the History of Present Illness to document this information.

7. Click in the **Quality** section to document that the patient describes the pain as an ache.

8. Click on the **Severity** section to document that the patient describes it as a 2 on a scale of 1–10.

9. Click on the **Duration** section to document 2 days.

10. To document the Review of Systems information, you will be clicking on the radio button next to sign/symptoms: **Yes** to indicate that the patient has that sign/symptom and **No** to indicate that they do not. Dr. Walden asks you to click **Yes** in the MS section—Injury. The **No** radio button can be clicked for all of the others.

11. Click the **Save** button.

Task 4.9 Complete Certificate to Return to Work or School

Mr. Ahmad's employer needs a certificate indicating that he is able to return to work after his injury. Dr. Walden has indicated that he is recovered enough from his injury to return to work without restrictions. She has asked you to complete the Certificate to Return to Work or School (refer to Task 2.7).

Now that Mr. Ahmad's visit is complete, the superbill and claim need to be completed (refer to Tasks 3.6 and 3.8). Using the information below, complete the Superbill to show the services provided and amount charged.

Diagnoses: Injury of left foot S99.922
Office Visit: 99212 $32.00
Copay: $10.00
Same Name as Patient
Same Address as Patient

---

1.   Click on the **Coding and Billing** module and locate Reuven Ahmad.
2.   From the list of **Encounters Not Coded,** click on the one you created today. This will open up the Superbill.
3.   On page 1 of the Superbill, you will enter the diagnosis by clicking on the **ICD-10** radio button and then entering **Injury of left foot S99.922**.
4.   In the **Office Visit** section, enter a **Rank** of **1** next to Problem focused, the fee of **$32.00** and the procedure code of **99212** in the Est column. Click **Save**.
5.   Click **Next** three times to get to page 4.
6.   Enter the **$10.00** in the **Copay** field.
7.   Enter **0.00** in the **Previous Balance** field and **32.00** in the **Balance Due** field.
8.   In the next section, click in the **Same Name as Patient** box and in the **Same Address as Patient** box.
9.   In the next section, click on the radio button for **Self** in the **Patient Relationship to Insured** area. Click in the **Married** box in the **Patient Status** area. Click the **No** radio button in the **Is there another health benefit plan?** area.
10. Enter **123-852-8523** in the Telephone section.
11. In the next section, click the **No** radio button for **Employment?, Auto Accident?,** and **Other Accident?**
12. Click in the **I am ready to submit the Superbill** box, then click the **Yes** radio button in the **Signature on file:** section and use today's date in the **Date** section.
13. Click the **Save** button and then click on the **Submit Superbill** button.
14. Select **Claim** from the information panel on the left side of the screen and perform a **Patient Search** for Reuven Ahmad. You will see the encounter for today with the status of Not Started. Click on the paper and pencil icon to open the claim.
15. The claim consists of seven tabs. Review the autopopulated information for the Patient Info, Provider Info, Payer Info, Encounter Notes, and Claim Info tabs. Add any missing information and click the **Save** button for each tab.
16. On the **Charge Capture** tab, enter today's date as the **DOS From** and **DOS To**.
17. Enter 99212 in the **CPT/HCPCS** column.
18. Click the Place of Service link to determine the correct the POS (Place of Service) code. Enter the correct code in the **POS** column.
19. Enter **1** in the **DX** column. This refers to ranking of the diagnosis found on the **Encounter Notes** page.
20. Enter **32.00** in the **Fee** column.
21. Enter **1** in the **Units** column.
22. Enter Click the **Save** button.
23. Click on the **Submission** tab and click the checkbox next to **I am ready to submit the Claim**.
24. Select the **Yes** radio button in the Signature on File field and enter **today's date** in the Date field.
25. Click the **Submit Claim** button.

Once again, you have quickly and efficiently learned new skills. You have also been able to apply the skills that you have learned previously. You are well on your way to being a fantastic medical assistant!

5. Day Five

Task 5.1 Updating Patient Demographics

Today Jill would like you to work in the billing department of the clinic. Correct billing is key to keeping the practice afloat financially. Attention to detail is especially important in this area.

You will start by updating demographics, creating a superbill, and then posting payments to patient ledgers. A patient ledger is where all financial activity for a patient is tracked. Any services or supplies that are given to a patient, any payments that are made, and any adjustments to the account are listed on the ledger, in which a running total of the account is kept.

People often move, change jobs, or change insurance carriers. All of these circumstances can impact billing. Patient statements need the correct patient address; insurance claims need the correct employer and insurance information. If the clinic does not have the correct information, billing can be delayed, which means there is a delay in reimbursement for the clinic. Jill has asked you to update the following patient demographic information.

Reuven Ahmad, DOB 09/12/1976, has been laid off by his employer. Reuven cannot afford to pay the insurance premium, even under COBRA, so he no longer has insurance.

1. Click on the **Patient Demographics** icon and perform a **Patient Search**.
2. Update the Guarantor and Insurance information (refer to Task 2.5).
3. Click the **Save Patient** button.

◎ PROFESSIONAL TIP

It is important to remain nonjudgmental when dealing with patients. When a patient has been laid off from his or her job and no longer has health insurance, they may feel bad about coming to the doctor. It is part of your job to make the patient feel as comfortable as possible in these circumstances. Having a list of community resources that may help is a good idea. The clinic may have a policy that will allow the patient to set up a payment plan to pay off the account over time. It is important to know the policies and procedures of the clinic when dealing with these sensitive situations.

Julia Berkley, DOB 07/05/1998, has moved to 125 1st Avenue, Anytown, AL 12345.

1. Click on the **Patient Demographics** icon and perform a **Patient Search**.
2. Update the appropriate fields.
3. Click the **Save Patient** button.

Quinton Brown, DOB 02/24/1986, now has insurance (Fig. 5.1).

1. Click on the **Patient Demographics** icon and perform a **Patient Search**.
2. Update the appropriate fields.
3. Click the **Save Patient** button.

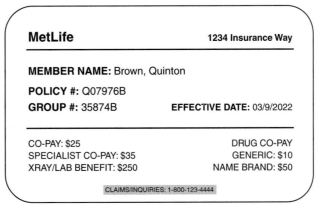

Figure 5.1 Quinton Brown's insurance card.

Task 5.2 Preparing a Superbill

Kyle Reeves, DOB 01/01/2004, has been seeing Dr. Angela Perez for an ongoing issue of upper abdominal pain and nausea. Today Kyle is here for an upper GI endoscopy with biopsies. Jill has asked you to complete the superbill for this procedure (refer to Task 3.6). Using the information below, complete the Superbill to show the services provided and amount charged for each. Before you can complete the Superbill, you will need to create an encounter in the Clinical Care module (see Task 2.9), before moving to the Coding and Billing module.

> Diagnoses: Upper abdominal pain, unspecified R10.10, Nausea R11.0
> Upper GI endoscopy with biopsy: 43239 $154.00
> Insured's Name: Kim Reeves
> Insured's Address: Same Address as Patient

1. Click on the **Clinical Care** module and perform a search to locate Kyle Reeves (DOB 01/01/2004). Click on the radio button next to his name and then click on the **Select** button.
2. To create an encounter, click on **Office Visit** in the Info Panel. If encounters already exist for Kyle, you will need to click on the **Add New** tab.
3. Select **Follow-up/Established Visit** for the Visit Type and **Angela Perez, MD** for the Provider and click on the **Save** button.
4. After the encounter has been created, click on the **Coding and Billing** module and locate Kyle Reeves.
5. From the list of **Encounters Not Coded,** click on the one you created today. This will open up the Superbill.
6. On page 1 of the Superbill, you will be entering the diagnosis by clicking on the ICD-10 radio button and then entering **Upper abdominal pain, unspecified R10.10** in the Rank 1 box, and **Nausea R11.0** in the Rank 2 box. Click **Save** and then click **Next** twice to get to page 3.
7. In the **Inpatient/Outpatient Procedure** section (on page 3 of the Superbill), enter a **Rank** of **1** next to Upper GI endoscopy w/biopsy, the fee of **$154.00** and the procedure code of **43239** in the Code column. Click **Save**.
8. Click **Next** to get to page 4.
9. Enter **25.00** in the **Copay** field.
10. Enter **0.00** in the **Previous Balance** field and **154.00** in the **Balance Due** field.
11. In the next section, enter **Kim Reeves** in the **Insured's Name** box and check the **Same Address as Patient** box.
12. In the next section, click on the radio button for **Child** in the **Patient Relationship to Insured** area. Click in the **Single** box in the **Patient Status** area. Click the **No** radio button in the **Is there another health benefit plan?** area.
13. Enter **123-225-6499** in the Telephone section.
14. In the next section click the **No** radio button for **Employment?**, **Auto Accident?**, and **Other Accident?**
15. Click in the **I am ready to submit the Superbill** box, then click the **Yes** radio button in the **Signature on file:** section and use today's date in the **Date:** section.
16. Click the **Save** button and then click on the **Submit Superbill** button.

Task 5.3 Posting Charges to a Ledger

Occasionally the clinic provides services that are not related to a medical condition. Charges for those services must be posted to the patient ledger.

Copying of Medical Records

Monique Jones, DOB 06/23/1993, is planning an extensive trip to Europe and would like to have a copy of her medical records with her just in case she needs them. It is the policy at the Walden-Martin Family Medical Clinic to charge for records that are not being released to another provider or to the court. There will be a $5.00 charge for the copying and sending of the records.

1. Click on the **Coding and Billing** tab and then select **Ledger** from the information panel on the left side of the screen. Perform a **Patient Search**.
2. Use today's date for the **Transaction Date** and **DOS**.
3. Enter Medical Records for the service and 5.00 in the **Charges** column..
4. Click the **Save** button.

Forms Completion

Daniel Miller, DOB 03/21/2021, is going to be attending a new daycare. This new facility requires that a form be completed by the physician. There is a $10.00 fee for this service.

1. Locate the patient's **Ledger**. Notice that the Guarantor for this account is Chris Miller. As Daniel is a minor, he is not legally responsible for the bill. The guarantor is his parent.
2. Using today's date, post the charges for the form completion service to Daniel's ledger.
3. Click the **Save** button.

Another important part of the billing process is sending out patient statements. A statement can serve two purposes: it can let the patient know which services were provided and the fee for those services, and it can notify the patient of how much he or she owes the clinic.

Because the two services provided above are not covered by insurance, Jill has asked you to generate statements for those services to be sent to the patients.

Statement for Monique Jones

1. Locate the **Patient Statement** in the **Form Repository** and perform a **Patient Search**.
2. Confirm the autopopulated fields.
3. Using today's date, complete the fields using Medical Records for the description. The full charge will be the patient's responsibility and should be paid in full by 1 month from today.
4. Click the **Save to Patient Record** button.

Statement for Daniel Miller

1. Complete the **Patient Statement** for Daniel.
2. Click the **Save to Patient Record** button.

On 01/26/2022, Erma Willis, DOB 12/09/1956, was seen by Dr. Kahn and had some skin lesions removed. Today the insurance payment has come through. The total charge for her visit on 01/26 was $107.58. Her insurance company has made a payment of 80%, or $86.06. This payment needs to be posted to her ledger.

1. Within the **Coding & Billing** tab, select **Ledger** form the left Info Panel.
2. Perform a Patient Search to locate Erma's ledger. Click on the radio button next to her name and then click on the **Select** button.
3. To open the ledger, click on the arrow to the right of Erma Willis's name. This will open up the ledger.
4. Click in the gray box under **Transaction Date** to open the calendar picker and choose today's date.
5. Click in the gray box under **DOS** (date of service) to open the calendar picker and choose 01/26/2022.
6. Select **David Kahn, MD** from the **Provider** drop-down menu.
7. Select **INSPYMT** from the **Service** drop-down menu.
8. Enter **86.06** in the **Payment** column.
9. Click the **Save** button.

Erma had received the explanation of benefits from her insurance company stating that she owed $21.74 for the skin lesion removals. She has sent a check for her portion and it has arrived today. This payment needs to be posted to her ledger.

1. Within the **Coding & Billing** tab, select **Ledger** form the left Info Panel.
2. Perform a Patient Search to locate Erma's ledger. Click on the radio button next to her name and then click on the **Select** button.
3. To open the ledger, click on the arrow to the right of Erma Willis's name. This will open up the ledger.
4. Click in the gray box under **Transaction Date** to open the calendar picker and choose today's date.
5. Click in the gray box under **DOS** (date of service) to open the calendar picker and choose 01/26/2022.
6. Select **David Kahn, MD** from the **Provider** drop-down menu.
7. Select **PTPYMTCK** from the **Service** drop-down menu.
8. Enter **21.74** in the **Payment** column.
9. Click the **Save** button.

Task 5.7 Completing a Day Sheet

The Day Sheet is used to track all of the services that were provided and all of the payments received in the clinic on a given day. All charges, payments, and adjustments are listed, along with the new balance on the patient account and the old balance (the balance prior to today's charges, payments, and/or adjustments) on the patient account. Jill has asked that you enter the following services and payments on the Day Sheet for today:

> Janine Butler: Services 99215 $75.00, 93000 $89.00; payment—check (Patient Payment Check [PTPYMTCK]) $25.00; old balance $346.00
>
> Robert Caudill: Services 99203 $70.00, 69210 $46.00; payment—cash (Patient Payment Cash [PTPYMTCSH]) $10.00; old balance $0.00
>
> Pedro Gomez: Services 99204 $89.00, 45330 $90.00; old balance $0.00
>
> Talibah Nasser: Services 99213 $43.00; payment—check (PTPYMTCK) $10.00; old balance $158.00
>
> Ella Rainwater: Services 99212 $32.00; old balance $35.00
>
> Kyle Reeves: Insurance payment (Insurance Payment [INSPYMT]) $120.00; adjustment $35.00; old balance $155.00
>
> Ken Thomas: Insurance payment (INSPYMT) $550.00; adjustment $120.00; old balance $820.00
>
> Erma Washington: Insurance payment (INSPYMT) $86.06; old balance $107.58
>
> Erma Washington: Payment – check (PTPYMNTCK) $21.74; old balance $21.74

Day Sheet Entries

When posting to the Day Sheet (Fig. 5.2), one line is typically used for each patient (with last name listed first), so you should list all services provided in the services area of the Day Sheet separated

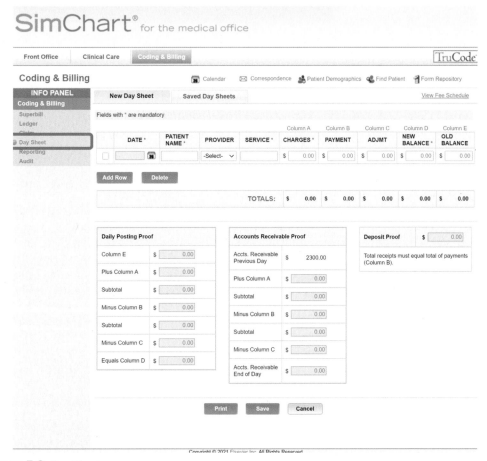

Figure 5.2 Day Sheet.

by a comma, that is, 99213, 81000, and the total of all services in the Charges column. For insurance payments, use the code INSPYMT in the Service column. You will have to calculate the new balance by starting with the old balance, adding in any charges and subtracting any payments and/or adjustments.

1. Click on the **Coding and Billing** tab to locate the **Day Sheet** on the left side.
2. Using the information provided above, enter all of the charges, payments, and adjustments for each patient on a separate line, using the **Add Row** button as needed.

Daily Proof of Posting; Accounts Receivable Proof

To verify that all of the numbers have been entered correctly, you will need to complete the Daily Posting Proof. The Accounts Receivable Proof provides the accounts receivable balance after the day's activities. This amount is carried forward to the next day's Day Sheet.

1. Using the column totals that have been autocalculated, complete the **Daily Posting Proof**. Your final total should match the total in Column D. If not, you will need to recheck the numbers entered into the Day Sheet. Make sure that your math was correct when adding the fees entered in the Charges column and when you calculated the New Balance.
2. Complete the **Accounts Receivable Proof**.
3. Enter the amount from Column B in the **Deposit Proof**. This number should match the amount of the Deposit Slip.
4. Click the **Save** button.

Task 5.8 Preparing the Bank Deposit Slip

At the end of the day, the last task in the business office is to prepare the bank deposit slip. All of the payments received for the day are listed on this slip. This slip, along with the endorsed checks and any cash received, are taken to the bank so that the funds can be deposited in the clinic's bank account.

Bank Deposit Slip

1. Click on the **Form Repository** icon and then **Office Forms** to locate the **Bank Deposit Slip**.
2. Use the payments listed in Task 5.7 to complete the bank deposit slip, listing the patient's last name first.
3. Click the **Save** button.

Jill is very impressed with your work in the billing department! She would like to you to continue to develop your scribing skills and has asked you to work with Dr. Walden as her scribe.

Task 5.9 Documenting Chief Complaint, History of Present Illness, Review of Systems, and Progress Notes

Janine Butler, DOB 04/25/1977, is here today to see Dr. Walden. Last night she went out to eat and, after taking just a couple bites of her lobster, developed swelling of the lips, tingling of the throat and mouth, and hives on her arms and chest. She quit eating the lobster and went home. This morning, most of her symptoms are gone, but she still has a few hives (refer to Task 2.9).

1. Click on the **Clinical Care** tab and locate Janine Butler's name in the List of Patients. Click on the radio button next to her name and then click on the **Select** button.
2. In order to enter the information into the EHR, you will need to create an encounter. Click on **Office Visit** in the Info Panel.
3. Select **Urgent Visit** for the Visit Type and **Julie Walden, MD** for the Provider and click on the **Save** button. At this time, the medical record will open up and the Record drop-down menu will appear.
4. Click on **Chief Complaint** from the Record drop-down menu.
5. Click in the textbox under **Chief Complaint**. Dr. Walden asks you to document the information provided by the patient about her experience last night in the Chief Complaint section. Remember to use quotation marks around statements that are in the patient's own words.
6. Dr. Walden then moves on to the **History of the Present Illness**. Document the information about the resolving hives.
7. To document the Review of Systems information, you will be clicking on the radio button next to sign/symptoms. Click **Yes** to indicate that the patient has that sign/symptom and **No** to indicate that they do not. Dr. Walden asks you to click Yes to **Rashes** in the **Hem/Skin** Section. The **No** radio button can be clicked for all of the others.
8. Click the **Save** button.
9. From the **Record** drop-down menu, select Progress Notes.
10. Dr. Walden asks you to document the symptoms that the patient described from the night before in the **Subjective** section.
11. Dr. Walden asks you to document "Resolving hives seen on the arms and chest." in the **Objective** section.
12. Dr. Walden asks you to document "Allergic reaction to shellfish." in the **Assessment** section.
13. Dr. Walden asks you to document "Allergy testing to be completed within the next month, patient instructed to avoid all shellfish." in the **Plan** section.
14. Click the **Save** button.

In addition to the progress notes, Dr. Walden has asked you to update Janine's allergy list to reflect the shellfish allergy.

1. While in the encounter created above, click on the **Record** drop-down menu and select **Allergies**.
2. Click on the **Add Allergy** button and click on the radio button next to **Food**.
3. Select **Shellfish** from the **Allergen** drop-down menu.
4. Check the box next to **Hives**.
5. Check the box next to **Other** and enter "Swelling of the lips and tingling of the mouth and throat."
6. Click the radio button next to **Mild** in the **Reaction Severity** section.
7. Click the radio button next to **Self** in the **Informant** section and the radio button next to **Very Reliable** in the **Confidence Level** section.
8. Click on the **Save** button.

Dr. Walden is very impressed with your scribing abilities and would like you to work with her again if you have time during your practicum.

You are halfway through your administrative practicum! You have accomplished so much in just 5 days. Give yourself a round of applause!

6. Day Six

You are back in the billing department today to learn more of what is involved in collecting funds for services rendered. One of those tasks is to send out collection letters for balances that have been outstanding for more than 60 days. It is the policy of the Walden-Martin Family Medical Clinic to give the patient 10 days to respond to a collection letter before further action is taken.

It has been discovered that Anna Richardson, DOB 02/14/1986, has an outstanding balance from DOS 01/21/2022. Her insurance made a payment, but there is still a balance due that is her responsibility. Jill asks that you create the collection letter for this account.

To complete the collection letter, you will need to determine which services were provided and what the balance is on Anna's account. That information can be found on the Superbill and Ledger.

1. Click on the **Coding and Billing** tab and gather the necessary information from the **Superbill** and **Ledger**.
2. Click on the **Correspondence** icon, **Letters**, and **Collection**. Perform a **Patient Search**.
3. Verify autopopulated information and enter the outstanding balance, the reason for the balance, date of service, and the date 10 days from today's date (for the Failure to respond before date).
4. Click on the **Save to Patient Record** button.

The balance left on an account after the insurance has paid is sometimes the patient's responsibility due to the deductible not being met yet, or coinsurance that is the patient's responsibility. Sometimes the balance is the patient's responsibility because the service has been denied by the insurance carrier. The patient may not realize that they are responsible for that balance. The Walden-Martin Family Medical Clinic has a policy of sending letters to patients when services have been denied by their carriers so that they are aware that it is their responsibility. It is also part of that policy to allow a patient 30 days from the date of the letter to pay the outstanding balance.

In reviewing the accounts with outstanding balances, it is discovered that Norma Washington, DOB 08/01/1953, has an outstanding balance for a Pap test performed on 03/24/2022. This service was denied by Medicare 2 weeks ago because Norma had a normal Pap test the previous year and Medicare pays for a screening Pap test only every 2 years. Jill asks that you create the denial letter for Norma Washington.

To complete the denial letter, you will need to determine the balance on Norma's account.

1. Determine the balance on the account by viewing the **Ledger**.
2. Select the **Denial** letter template from the information panel on the left side of the screen and perform a **Patient Search**.
3. Verify the autopopulated information and enter the date of service, date of claim denial, the service that was denied, reason for denial, the outstanding balance, and the payment due date.
4. Click on the **Save to Patient Record** button.

The majority of the income for any medical clinic comes from insurance reimbursement. It is important that all claims are paid in a timely fashion. To be sure that happens, the medical clinic must keep track of claims and follow up on those that are not paid in the expected time frame (10–14 days for an electronic claim, 30–45 days for a paper claim). If a claim is not paid in the expected time frame, an Insurance Claims Tracer can be used to follow up with the insurance carrier.

It has been discovered that a claim for Truong Tran, DOB 05/30/2000, for DOS 02/16/2022 has not been paid or denied. Jill asks that you prepare the Insurance Claims Tracer form for claim #133781.

To complete this form, you will need the following information from the original claim:

Information needed:	Location:
Insurance carrier	Payer info tab
Date of Service	Encounter notes tab
Diagnosis	Encounter notes tab
Procedure code	Charge capture tab
Procedure cost	Charge capture tab

1. Locate the **Insurance Claims Tracer** in the **Form Repository** and perform a **Patient Search**.
2. Confirm the autopopulated fields.
3. Enter the information that was collected from the original claim in the appropriate fields, including the claim # of 133781.
4. Click the **Save to Patient Record** button.

Task 6.4 Maintaining a Petty Cash Fund

Petty cash is a small amount of cash kept on hand to cover some of the everyday expenses that arise, such as parking, postage, or lunch for the doctor. While the name "petty cash" may lead you to believe that it is not very important, that would be an incorrect assumption. It is important to keep track of how those funds are used and to make sure that there is actual cash in the petty cash fund for those minor expenses. Due to a turnover in staff at the Walden-Martin Family Medical Clinic, the petty cash fund has not been well managed lately. Jill asks that you take on that task to update it.

When you open the lockbox that is used for the petty cash fund, you see that there are some receipts and $200 in cash. You also notice that no one has recorded anything in the petty cash journal (Fig. 6.1) for last month. Your first step is to organize the receipts by date and then start the petty cash journal for last month.

> Dated the 18th, receipt for tissues and cotton balls purchased from the drug store, $15.89
> Dated the 4th, receipt for postage due paid, $4.75
> Dated the 26th, receipt for lunch for the doctor, $12.50
> Dated the 12th, receipt for parking for a conference attended by the office manager in another city, $6.50

1. Locate the **Petty Cash Journal** form in the **Office Forms** section of the **Form Repository**.
2. Using the information provided above, post the items to the Petty Cash Journal, entering the dollar amounts in the correct column, using the **Add Row** button as needed. (Remember that all fields with an asterisk [*] are mandatory.)

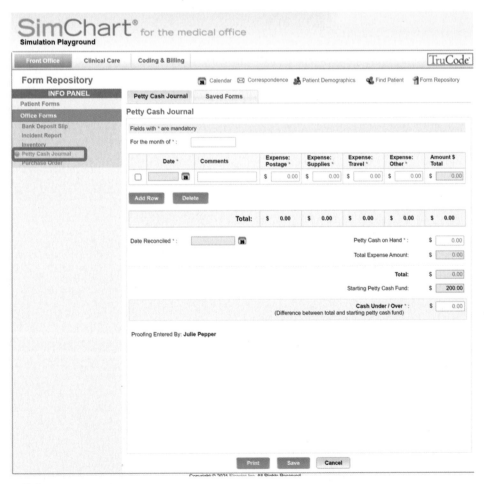

Figure 6.1 Petty Cash Journal.

3. Complete all other required fields, using today's date as the **Date Reconciled**.
4. Click the **Save** button.

You have had a couple of busy days in the billing department. You should now have a better understanding of how the billing process works to keep the money coming into the practice. You should also have a better understanding of how important it is to pay attention to the details. If you are off by one number, it can impact many areas of the reimbursement cycle.

There are number of different forms that are used in a medical office and Jill would like you to get familiar with some more of those forms. The rest of your tasks today will involve various forms for patients and for office supplies.

Often a requisition form needs to be completed for services provided to patients. The requisition indicates exactly what services are needed, along with diagnosis codes for those services. The next two tasks will involve creating requisitions.

Task 6.5 Requisition for a Mammogram

Dr. Perez has just finished an annual physical with Noemi Rodiguez, DOB 11/4/1980. Ms. Rodriquez has a family history of breast cancer and Dr. Perez discussed the option of starting annual mammograms. Ms. Rodriquez likes that plan and Dr. Perez has asked you to complete the requisition for a bilateral mammogram. Using the following information, complete the requisition form:

> Insurance Co: Aetna
> Ordering Physician: Angela N. Perez, MD
> Diagnosis: Family history of malignant neoplasm of breast
> Diagnosis Code: Z80.3

1. Click on the **Forms Repository** icon and the select **Requisition** from the left Info Panel (Fig. 6.2).
2. Select **Radiology** from the Requisition Type drop-down menu (Fig. 6.2).
3. Click on the **Patient Search** button to locate Noemi Rodriguez.
4. Enter the date for Tuesday of next week in **Service Date** field.
5. Enter Angela N. Perez, MD in the **Ordering Physician** field.
6. Document the **Diagnosis** as given above.
7. Document the **Diagnosis Code** as given above.
8. In the **Women's Imaging** section, check the box next to **Screening Mammogram**.
9. Click the **No** radio button for **History of Kidney Problems**, **Contrast Allergy**, and **Is the patient on anticoagulants?**
10. Click on the **Routine** radio button for **Exam is**.
11. Click on the **Save to Patient Record** button.

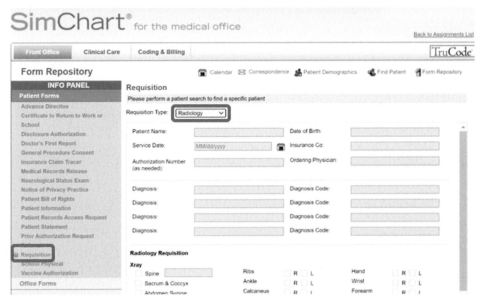

Figure 6.2 Radiology Requisition.

Task 6.6 Requisition for a Transesophageal Echo (TEE)

Dr. Kahn is seeing Robert Caudill, DOB 10/31/1940, today. Mr. Caudill called in this morning complaining of fatigue, shortness of breath, and he says it feels like his heart is fluttering in his chest. Dr. Kahn suspects that Mr. Caudill has atrial fibrillation and would like him to have a transesophageal echo (TEE) today. Using the procedure used in Task 6.5 and the following information, enter the requisition:

Insurance Co: Medicare
Ordering Physician: David Kahn, MD
Diagnosis: Fatigue
Diagnosis Code: R53.83
Diagnosis: Irregular heartbeat
Diagnosis Code: I49.9
Diagnosis: Flutter
Diagnosis Code: I49.8
Diagnosis: Shortness of breath
Diagnosis Code: R06.02

Maria Gomez has called because Pedro, DOB 07/01/2016, will be changing schools and the new school has requested a new school physical form be completed. She will be stopping in to pick it up tomorrow. Using the information below, complete the school physical form for Pedro Gomez:

> It is Walden-Martin's policy to attach an Immunization transcript to the school physical forms.
>   No need to complete the Immunization section of the form.
> Pedro's last physical was 3 months ago
> Height: 50.4 inches, Weight 56.5 pounds, BMI 13.6, BP 96/64
> No conditions or disabilities that would affect behavior at school
> No allergies
> No epinephrine auto-injector required
> No treatment plan
> No medications
> Lead screening is complaint
> Can participate in PE without restrictions
> Passed hearing screening; Comprehensive Exam Date same as physical exam date
> Passed vision screening; Comprehensive Exam Date same as physical exam date
> Passed scoliosis screening; Comprehensive Exam Date same as physical exam date

1. Click on the **Forms Repository** icon and the select **School Physical** from the left Info Panel (Fig. 6.3).
2. Click on the **Patient Search** button to locate Pedro Gomez.
3. Using the information provided, complete the form.
4. In the **Health Care Provider Signature** area, enter today's date in the **Date** field.
5. Click on the **Save to Patient Record** button.

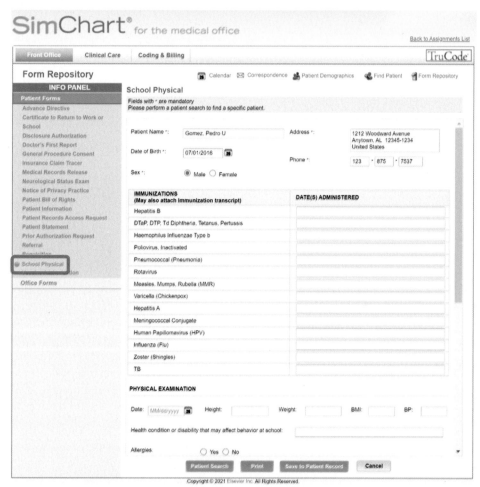

Figure 6.3 School Physical.

Task 6.8 Vaccine Authorization

Johnny Parker, DOB 6/15/2019, is in today to get his influenza vaccine. Jean Burke, NP, has asked you complete the Vaccine Authorization form so that Johnny's mother can sign it. Using the information below, complete the form:

> Johnny is not sick and does not have a fever
> Johnny is not allergic to chicken, eggs, or egg products
> Johnny has not had an allergic reaction to any previous injections
> Johnny is not pregnant
> Johnny does not have a clotting disorder, and is not taking blood thinning medication

1. Click on the **Forms Repository** icon and the select **Vaccine Authorization** from the left Info Panel (Fig. 6.4).
2. Click on the **Patient Search** button to locate Johnny Parker.
3. Using the information provided, complete the form.
4. Click on the **Save to Patient Record** button.

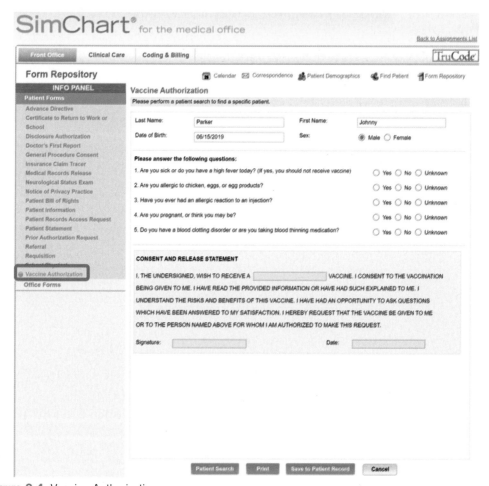

Figure 6.4 Vaccine Authorization.

Amma Patel, DOB 1/14/1996, is in today because she has been having some significant bleeding between periods. After her examination and reviewing the test results, Dr. Walden is recommending a D&C (dilatation and curettage). Ms. Patel and Dr. Walden agree that this is the best treatment, and Dr. Walden asks you to prepare the general procedure consent form. Use the following information to complete the form:

> Date – use today's date
> Condition – Menorrhagia
> Procedure proposed – Dilatation and Curettage (D&C)

1. Click on the **Forms Repository** icon and the select **General Procedure Consent** from the left Info Panel (Fig. 6.5).
2. Click on the **Patient Search** button to locate Amma Patel.
3. Using the information provided complete the form.
4. Click on the **Save to Patient Record** button.

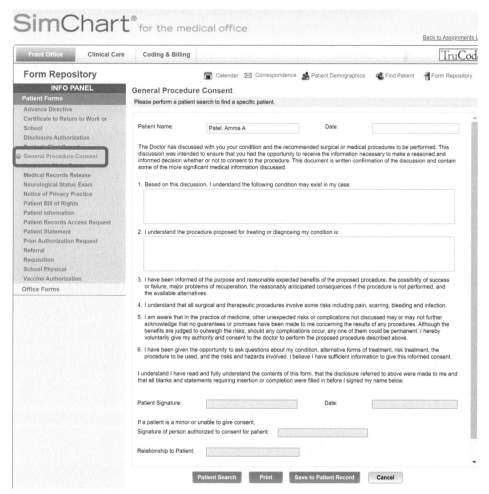

Figure 6.5 General Procedure Consent.

Task 6.10 Purchase Order

For your last task today, Jill would like you to complete a purchase order for the supplies that are needed. Using the list below, complete the Purchase Order form.

The supplier is McKesson (123-123-4579) and the PO Number is S00425662. Use the information collected below to complete the Inventory form and determine the supplies needed based on the Quantity on Hand and the Reorder Levels. Then use this information to complete a Purchase Order.

Table paper, Unit – Case/12, Quantity to Reorder – 5, Price/Unit - $49.19
Alcohol prep pads, Unit – Box/200, Quantity to Reorder – 20, Price/Unit - $3.3
Sterile 4×4 gauze squares, Unit – Box/100, Quantity to Reorder – 30, Price/Unit - $30.69
25 G × 5/8" 3cc syringes, Unit – Box/100, Quantity to Reorder – 10, Price/Unit - $73.89
Nitrile powder-free exam gloves, Unit – Box/100, Quantity to Reorder – 20, Price/Unit - $12.49
Surpass facial tissues, Unit – Case/30, Manufacturer – Quantity to Reorder – 4, Price/Unit – $52.89

---

1. Click on the **Forms Repository** icon and under **Office Forms** in the left Info Panel, select **Purchase Order** (Fig. 6.6).
2. Document your name in the **Submitter** field.
3. Document **S00425662** in the **PO Number** field.

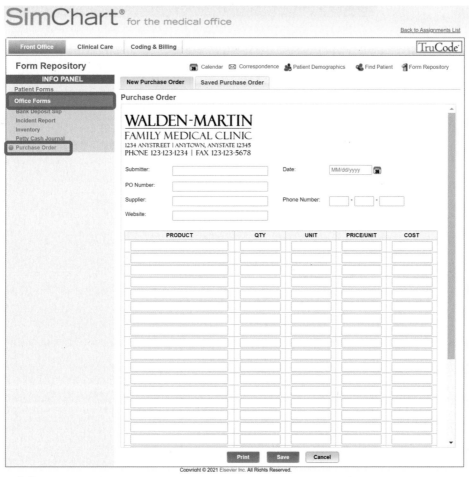

Figure 6.6 Purchase Order.

4. Document today's date in the **Date** field.
5. Document **McKesson** in the **Supplier** field.
6. Document **123-123-4579** in the **Phone Number** field.
7. Document **Table paper** in the **Product** column.
8. Document **5** in the **Quantity** column.
9. Document **case** in the **Unit** column.
10. Document **49.19** in the Price/**Unit** column.
11. Document **245.95** (5x 49.19)in the **Cost** column.
12. Continue adding items to the purchase order following the steps above.
13. Click the **Save** button.

You have been doing a great job. Keep up the good work!

7. Day Seven

Today Jill has given you some tasks to complete that are similar to tasks you have done before. For the scheduling tasks, Jill feels that you should be familiar enough with the process that she has given you just some basic information.

Task 7.1 Establishing a Meeting

Your first task for today is to schedule a meeting for all three of the providers to discuss equipment purchases for the coming year. They would like the meeting to occur next week in the afternoon. You will then send a memorandum to all the providers, telling them the date and time of the meeting.

Scheduling the Meeting

1. Use the arrow keys on the **Calendar** to move to next week.
2. Locate a day and time, after lunch, when all three providers are available for 1 hour.
3. Schedule a **Block** appointment for all providers.
4. Click on the **Save** button.

Creating the Memorandum

1. Locate the **Email Memorandum** template in Correspondence.
2. The Memorandum is being sent to Dr. Walden, Dr. Martin, and Jean Burke, NP.
3. Complete all fields and compose a professional message containing all of the information about the meeting.
4. Click on the **Save** button.

 PROFESSIONALISM

With so much of our personal communication happening in the electronic world, it is easy to let some of that style creep into our professional lives as well. It is important to keep electronic communication at work professional. Spelling and grammar are key components to professional communication. All words should be completely spelled out unless it is an accepted abbreviation. That means that "are" is spelled "are," not "R"; "you" is not "U"; and so on. If you are unsure about the spelling or grammar when sending an email, you can use the spell and grammar checker found in the email program or type it into a word processing program first. One caution, though: you should not rely solely on the spell-checker, as it will tell you only if the word is spelled incorrectly, not whether you have used it incorrectly; for example, to, too, and two are spelled correctly but have different meanings.

Task 7.2 Scheduling a Recurring Staff Meeting With a Memorandum

The providers at the Walden-Martin Family Medical Clinic feel that it is important to bring the staff together for a meeting once a month to disseminate important information about changes or new policies within the clinic, discuss any issues that may have come up, and provide an opportunity for the staff to come together as a team. A memorandum needs to be sent to all of the staff, telling them the day and time for the monthly meeting.

Scheduling a Recurring Meeting

Due to the providers' other commitments, such as hospital rounds, the meeting will need to be on Tuesdays at 2:00 PM. The only room large enough for all the staff to meet in is the Meeting Room.

1. Locate next Tuesday on the **Calendar**.
2. Create the monthly recurring appointment in the **Meeting Room**.
3. Click on the **Save** button.

Creating the Memorandum

1. Locate the **Email Memorandum** template in Correspondence.
2. The memorandum is being sent to **All Staff**.
3. Complete all fields and compose a professional message containing all of the information about the meeting.
4. Click on the **Save** button.

Task 7.3 Scheduling Office Procedures

There are several different office procedures that are done frequently at the Walden-Martin Family Medical Clinic. One procedure is a sigmoidoscopy, which takes 1 hour and is performed in Exam Room 1; another is a colposcopy, which takes 45 minutes and is performed in Exam Room 2. Dr. Martin has asked you to schedule one of his patients for a sigmoidoscopy, and Jean Burke, NP, has asked you to schedule one of her patients for a colposcopy with biopsy.

Charles Johnson, DOB 03/03/1966, needs to have a sigmoidoscopy scheduled. He is Dr. Martin's patient and would like to have this procedure done sometime next week when he can get an afternoon appointment.

1. Schedule Charles for the sigmoidoscopy procedure, making sure to designate the correct exam room and time for this procedure.

Noemi Rodriguez, DOB 11/04/1980, needs to have a colposcopy with biopsies scheduled. She is a patient of Jean Burke, NP, and would like to have this done as early in the day as possible on Thursday of next week.

1. Schedule Noemi for the colposcopy procedure, making sure to designate the correct exam room and time for this procedure.

Charles's insurance requires prior authorization for a sigmoidoscopy. Complete the appropriate form to request the prior authorization.

1. Locate the **Prior Authorization Request** form in the **Form Repository** and perform a patient search.
2. Use the information below to complete the form.
3. Click the **Save to Patient Record** button.

Ordering physician: James A. Martin
Provider contact name: Jill King
Place of service/treatment and address:
Walden-Martin Family Medical Clinic
1234 Anystreet
Anytown, AL 12345
Service requested: Sigmoidoscopy
Diagnosis/ICD code: Screening for malignant neoplasm of colon; ICD-10 Z12.11
Procedure/CPT code: 45330
Injury related?: No
Workers' Compensation related: No

Noemi's insurance also requires a prior authorization for a colposcopy. Complete the appropriate form to request the prior authorization.

1. Locate the **Prior Authorization Request** form and perform a **Patient Search**.
2. Use the information below to complete the form.
3. Click the **Save to Patient Record** button.

Ordering physician: Jean Burke, NP
Provider contact name: Jill King
Place of service/treatment and address:
Walden-Martin Family Medical Clinic
1234 Anystreet
Anytown, AL 12345
Service requested: Colposcopy with biopsies
Diagnosis/ICD code: Cervical intraepithelial neoplasm II; ICD-10 N87.1
Injury related?: No
Workers' Compensation related: No

Task 7.5 Scheduling Audiometry and Tympanometry

James Brown has called in because he is concerned about his daughter's hearing. Christina, DOB 8/3/2017, has had issues with chronic ear infections since she was quite young and is now not responding to her dad when he speaks to her, and her teacher has mentioned that Christina seems to be having some issue with hearing in class. Dr. Perez would like Christina to come in for audiometry and tympanometry today. Due to the need for specialized equipment and a soundproof room, these tests are done in Exam Room 7 and will take 1 hour to perform.

1. Schedule Christina for audiometry and tympanometry in the first available appointment this afternoon, making sure to designate the correct exam room and time for this procedure.

Task 7.6 Complete Superbill and Claim Form

Christina Brown has been seen, and her audiometry and tympanometry have been completed. Jill would like you to complete the Superbill and Claim Form using the information below. You will first have to create an encounter in the Clinical Care tab.

Diagnosis: ICD-10-CM Z01.100 Examination of ears and hearing without abnormal findings
Services Provided:
- Audiometry; Code – 92551, Fee $32.00
- Tympanometry; Code – 92567, Fee $248.57
- Insured Name: James Brown
- Insured Address: Same Address as Patient
- Patient Relationship to Insured: Child
- No other health plan
- Telephone: 123-456-1237
- Patient's condition is not related to employment, auto accident, or other accident.
- Signature on file with today's date

Kyle Reeves, DOB 01/01/2004, has called in because he has cut his finger and thinks he needs stitches. Schedule Kyle for the first available appointment for today (refer to Task 2.4). Because this is an urgent situation, you should try to schedule this with Kyle's usual provider, Julie Walden, MD, but if she is not available, Kyle should be scheduled with another provider.

Ken Thomas, DOB 10/25/1970, has emailed the clinic and is wondering what the cost of having a vasectomy is. He has requested a reply via email. Jill would like you to look up the fee for this procedure and then compose a professional email reply.

Fee Schedule

1. Click on the **Coding and Billing** tab to locate the link for the **Fee Schedule**.
2. Click on the link titled **Fee Schedule**.
3. Locate **Vasectomy** under **Office Procedures** and determine the fee.

Email

1. Find the **Blank Email** template by clicking on **Correspondence** and then perform a **Patient Search**.
2. Review the autopopulated fields and complete all other fields.
3. Compose a professional email, stating the fee for the requested procedure.
4. Click the **Send** button, and a copy of the email will be saved to the patient record.

 PROFESSIONALISM

Always keep in mind that you represent the clinic and providers for whom you work when you communicate with patients. The language used in an email to a patient should be as professional as the language you use to communicate with physicians and coworkers. Remember to use correct spelling and grammar. It is also important to remember to include a salutation and complimentary closing in a professional email.

Celia Tapia, DOB 05/18/1979, a patient of Dr. Martin, has missed several appointments and is not responding to phone messages left for her. Jill explains that it is the policy of the Walden-Martin Family Medical Clinic to terminate the physician/patient contract when more than three appointments have been missed and there is no response from the patient. She asks you to create the Patient Termination letter to be sent to Celia.

Creating the Letter

1. Locate the **Patient Termination** letter template in **Correspondence** and do a **Patient Search**.
2. Review the autopopulated fields and verify that the date of termination is 30 days from today's date.
3. Click the **Save to Patient Record** button.

Dr. Martin has been treating Ella Rainwater, DOB 07/11/1968, for type 2 diabetes mellitus. Ella has been having trouble keeping her blood glucose levels in control and Dr. Martin thinks she should see an endocrinologist, Dr. Randall Gilbert. Using the information below, complete the Medical Release form (refer to Task 2.8) so that Dr. Gilbert will have Ella's records for her appointment, which has been scheduled for 2 weeks from today. Walden-Martin Family Medical Clinic will be releasing all records.

New Provider:
Gilbert and Sullivan Endocrinology Clinic
922 Sugar Lane
Anytown, AL 12345-1234
Phone: 555-123-1886
Fax: 555-123-1314
Expiration date: 1 year from today

You have successfully completed your seventh day! You have learned much and are now applying it to new situations. You are using your critical thinking skills well.

8. Day Eight

To keep an office running smoothly and efficiently, there needs to be an adequate amount of supplies on hand to accomplish the tasks for the day. Inventory management is how an office knows when supplies are running low and when an order should be placed. Most offices make an inventory and order supplies on a set schedule. Some supplies may be ordered weekly and others may be ordered monthly or even quarterly. Jill would like you to take a look at the recent inventory that was made for the front office supplies and complete the inventory form. This information will be used to determine which supplies need to be ordered.

Table 8.1 shows the list of supplies with the quantity that is on hand. The reorder level is the point at which you need to order that particular supply. If there are seven of a particular item on hand and the reorder level is 10, that would indicate that you need to order more of that item. The quantity to reorder is how much of that supply should be ordered. You should order the full number of items listed in the quantity to reorder even though you still have some on hand. The number of items on hand should keep you supplied until the new order arrives.

Inventory Form

1. Locate the Inventory form in the Form Repository under Office Forms.
2. Using the information in Table 8.1, complete the form, using the Add button as needed to create additional rows.
3. Click the Save button.

Purchase Order

1. Determine which supplies need to be ordered based on the quantity on hand and the reorder level listed in Table 8.1. If the quantity on hand is at or below the reorder level, it should be ordered.
2. Locate the **Purchase Order** form in the **Form Repository** under **Office Forms** and print the blank form by clicking on the printer icon in the gray bar at the top of the form.

TABLE **8.1**

Supply List

	Quantity on Hand	Unit	Price/Unit	Reorder Levels	Quantity to Reorder
Jumbo paper clips, smooth	4 boxes	box	$1.10	5 boxes	20 boxes
Staples, ¼ in.	5 boxes	box	$3.79	7 boxes	30 boxes
White-out correction fluid, 3/pack	4 bottles	pack	$3.99	2 packs	15 packs
Manila end tab file folders, letter size, 100/box	3 boxes	box	$17.99	2 boxes	25 boxes
Print or write multiuse ID labels, 3 in. H×4 in. L, 80/pack	1 pack	pack	$6.99	1.5 pack	12 packs
AA alkaline batteries, 4/pack	6 each	pack	$4.99	1 pack	15 packs
3 in. × 5 in. line-ruled colored sticky notes, 5/pack	18 each	pack	$12.69	3 packs	2 packs
Paper clips, #1 size, nonskid	4.5 packs	pack	$6.14	5 packs	50 packs
Ballpoint pens, medium, black, dozen	11 each	dozen	$6.89	1 dozen	75 boxes

3. Using today's date and the information below, complete the top portion of the form.

> Submitter: Walden-Martin Family Medical Clinic
> PO number: 487762
> Supplier: Anytown Office Supply
> Phone: 123-123-9876
> Website: www.anytownofficesupply.com

4. List the items you have determined should be ordered, including the quantity, unit, and price/unit.
5. Calculate the cost of ordering that item by multiplying the quantity by the price/unit and enter this amount in the **Cost** column.
6. When all of the items have been listed, add up the cost of each item to determine the total cost of the order and enter this amount in the **Total** field.

Walter Biller, DOB 01/04/1978, a patient of Dr. Walden, needs to provide his employer with documentation that he is able to return to work after having broken his shoulder. It has been 8 weeks since the fracture, and Dr. Walden feels that he is completely healed and can return to work with no restrictions.

Complete the Certificate to Return to Work or School Form

1. Locate the Certificate to Return to Work or School form in the Form Repository and do a Patient Search.
2. Review the autopopulated field and complete the other fields using the information provided above.
3. Click on the Save to Patient Record button.

There have been some issues with employees at the Walden-Martin Family Medical Clinic using their cell phones during the workday. Some of the patients have noticed it and commented on it to Dr. Walden. Dr. Walden brought it to Jill's attention, and she has asked you to prepare a memorandum using today's date from Jill King, Office Manager, to all employees about the policy regarding the use of cell phones during working hours. The memorandum should remind the staff that cell phones should not be answered during working hours except in the case of emergencies. Staff can carry their cell phones with them, but they must be switched to silent mode. Cell phones should not be answered when working with patients. Texting and other cell phone activities should be limited to breaks and lunch times.

1. Locate the **Memorandum** template from the **Email** section of **Correspondence** and create a professional email to all employees reminding them of the cell phone policy.

 PROFESSIONALISM

In healthcare, it is important to keep things concise. This is true for professional correspondence as well as documentation in the health record. Your message should be clear and concise. Get to the point so you are not wasting anyone's time.

2. Click the **Send** button. A copy of the email will be saved and can be accessed by clicking on **Sent Memorandums**.

While you are working at the front desk, one of your duties is to handle any patient issues that come up. One of the most common situations that comes up is the walk-in patient, a patient who does not have an appointment scheduled and wants to be seen today. Some patients should be seen on the same day if possible, such as those who have a fever, sore throat, or painful urination; others can wait until the next available time slot such as an annual examination or wellness visit.

Annual Examination

Jeffrey Raymond, DOB 09/25/1960, stops by the Walden-Martin Family Medical Clinic. He has heard fantastic things about Dr. Walden and would like to schedule an annual exam with her, today if possible. You ask Jeffrey to complete a patient registration form while you view the schedule.

1. Locate Dr. Walden's schedule and find the next available time slot for an annual exam (45 minutes).
2. Jeffrey agrees to the date and time that you have found, so you schedule his appointment.
3. Using the completed **Patient Information** form (Fig. 8.1), fully complete the patient demographics section.

Fever and Sore Throat

Kay Peterson, DOB 08/06/1982, states that she has had a fever and sore throat for the past 2 days and really does not feel well. She is willing to see any provider if she can get an appointment today. You check the policy manual and you see that a fever and sore throat is listed under the conditions that should get a same-day appointment, even if it means double booking a provider. You have Kay complete a patient information form while you review the schedule.

1. Review the schedule and find the first available time slot (45 minutes) in today's schedule.
2. Kay agrees to the time you have available, so you schedule her appointment.
3. Using the completed **Patient Information** form (Fig. 8.2), fully complete the patient demographics section.

WALDEN-MARTIN
FAMILY MEDICAL CLINIC
1234 ANYSTREET | ANYTOWN, ANYSTATE 12345
PHONE 123-123-1234 | FAX 123-123-5678

PATIENT INFORMATION

First Name	MI	Last Name	Date of Birth	Sex
Jeffrey	S	Raymond	9/25/1969	M

SSN	Home Phone	Work Phone	Cell
987-23-5432	123-123-0449		

Home Address	City	State	Zip
916 Livingston Ln	Anytown	AL	12345

Marital Status	Employer	Driver's License #

Emergency Contact	Relationship to Patient	Phone Number
Julie Raymond		

RESPONSIBLE PARTY INFORMATION   **SELF** ☐

First Name	MI	Last Name	Date of Birth	Sex
Dr. Walden				

SSN	Home Phone	Work Phone	Cell
	123-123-1234		

Home Address	City	State	Zip
1234 Anystreet	Anytown	AL	12345

Employer		Relationship to Patient
Smith Electric		Self

INSURANCE INFORMATION

Primary Insurance Carrier	Phone Number
Met Life	800-123-4444

Address	City	State	Zip
1234 Insurance Ave	Anytown	AL	12345

Policy Holder Name (if different from patient)	Phone	Date of Birth	Sex
Julie Raymond	123-251-9686		

Policy Number	Group Number
L85027C	40275M

Secondary Insurance Carrier	Phone Number

Address	City	State	Zip

Policy Holder Name (if different from patient)	Phone	Date of Birth	Sex

Policy Number	Group Number

I hereby give lifetime authorization for payment of insurance benefits to be made directly to Walden-Martin Medical Group, and any assisting physicians, for services rendered. I understand that I am financially responsible for all charges whether or not they are covered by insurance. In the event of default, I agree to pay all costs of collection, and reasonable attorney's fees. I hereby authorize this healthcare provider to release all information necessary to secure the payment of benefits. I further agree that a photocopy of this agreement shall be as valid as the original.

Signature *JS Raymond*	Date

Figure 8.1 Jeffrey Raymond's Patient Information form.

WALDEN-MARTIN
FAMILY MEDICAL CLINIC
1234 ANYSTREET | ANYTOWN, ANYSTATE 1234
PHONE 123-123-1234 | FAX 123-123-5678

PATIENT INFORMATION

First Name	MI	Last Name		Date of Birth	Sex
Kay	M	Peterson		08/06/1991	F

SSN	Home Phone	Work Phone		Cell
123-45-9876	123-123-6798			

Home Address	City	State	Zip
916 Livingston Ln	Anytown	AL	12345-1234

Marital Status	Employer	Driver's License #
		AL535311

Emergency Contact	Relationship to Patient	Phone Number
Cathy Peterson		123-123-5421

RESPONSIBLE PARTY INFORMATION   SELF ☐

First Name	MI	Last Name	Date of Birth	Sex
Dr. Walden				

SSN	Home Phone	Work Phone	Cell
		123-123-4501	123-123-6667

Home Address	City	State	Zip
1234 Anystreet	Anytown	AL	12345

Employer		Relationship to Patient
Anytown Library		Self

INSURANCE INFORMATION

Primary Insurance Carrier	Phone Number
Aetna	800-123-2222

Address	City	State	Zip
1234 Insurance Way	Anytown	AL	12345

Policy Holder Name (if different from patient)	Phone	Date of Birth	Sex
Kay Peterson	123-251-9686		

Policy Number	Group Number	
824892N	42856M	

Secondary Insurance Carrier	Phone Number

Address	City	State	Zip

Policy Holder Name (if different from patient)	Phone	Date of Birth	Sex

Policy Number	Group Number	

I hereby give lifetime authorization for payment of insurance benefits to be made directly to Walden-Martin Medical Group, and any assisting physicians, for services rendered. I understand that I am financially responsible for all charges whether or not they are covered by insurance. In the event of default, I agree to pay all costs of collection, and reasonable attorney's fees. I hereby authorize this healthcare provider to release all information necessary to secure the payment of benefits. I further agree that a photocopy of this agreement shall be as valid as the original.

Signature *Kay Peterson*	Date

Figure 8.2 Kay Peterson's Patient Information form.

Task 8.5 Telephone Messages

Locate the "Telephone Messages" area on the companion Evolve website (Task 8.5). These are the nonurgent messages that came into the clinic over the lunch hour. Jill would like you to listen to the messages, complete a Phone Message for each in the electronic health record, schedule appointments (if necessary), and respond to the patient.

 PROFESSIONALISM

Phone messages can be left for a number of different reasons: medical questions for the physicians; requests for procedures, lab results, or prescription refills; billing questions; or general questions. Some of these can be handled by the medical assistant, such as general billing questions, directions to the clinic, or scheduling appointments, but some need to be handled by the provider, such as questions regarding care and treatment, requests for new prescriptions, or complications from a procedure. If you are unsure whether you can take care of the situation, ask your supervisor.

Document Phone Message, Schedule Appointment, Email Patient

1. Locate Phone Messages in Correspondence and perform a Patient Search.
2. Document the information accurately.
3. If necessary, schedule the appointment as close as possible to the time requested by the patient. Indicate the date and time of the appointment in the Action Documentation section of the Phone Message.
4. Click the Save to Patient Record button.
5. If an appointment has been scheduled, use the template to compose a professional email indicating the date and time the appointment has been scheduled for, which doctor it is scheduled with, and how the patient should contact the office to change the appointment if the time is inconvenient.

 PROFESSIONALISM

Email correspondence and interoffice messaging are often used to communicate within the medical clinic. It is important to maintain patient confidentiality in all correspondence. It may be the policy to use only a patient identification number in correspondence within the clinic. You should be knowledgeable of the clinic's policies regarding email communication.

6. Click the **Send** button. You can view the email by clicking on the **Find Patient** icon, performing a **Patient Search**, and then scrolling down to the **Correspondence** section.
   Complete these steps for all messages remaining for this task.
   Jill would like you to continue to develop your scribing skills. She recognizes that the need for scribes is growing and will continue to grow for the foreseeable future. She wants you to be well prepared to take on this role when you have completed your education. To help with that she would like you to work with Dr. Perez as her scribe.
   Maude Crawford, DOB 12/22/1955, has recently signed up for Medicare Part B. Medicare Part B covers a "Welcome to Medicare" preventive visit once within the first 12 months of signing up for Part B. For this visit Mrs. Crawford will not be responsible for any of the expense and the Part B deductible does not apply. This wellness visit includes:
   - Certain screenings, flu and pneumococcal shots, and referral for other care, if needed
   - Height, weight, and blood pressure measurements
   - A calculation of body mass index
   - A simple vision test
   - A review of your potential risk for depression and your level of safety
   - An offer to talk with you about creating advance directives
   The remaining tasks for today will have you scribing the various aspects of a "Welcome to Medicare" wellness visit.

Task 8.6 Documenting Chief Complaint, History of Present Illness, and Review of Systems

As with most visits, a "Welcome to Medicare" visit will start with documenting the chief complaint, history of present illness and review of systems (refer to Task 2.9).

1. Click on the **Clinical Care** tab and locate Maude Crawford's name in the List of Patients. Click on the radio button next to her name and then click on the **Select** button.
2. In order to enter the information into the EHR you will need to create an encounter. Click on **Office Visit** in the Info Panel.
3. Select **Wellness Exam** for the Visit Type and **Angela N. Perez, MD** for the Provider and click on the **Save** button. At this time, the medical record will open up and **Record** drop-down menu will appear.
4. Click on **Chief Complaint** from the **Record** drop-down menu.
5. Click in the textbox under **Chief Complaint**. Dr. Perez asks you to document that Mrs. Crawford is here for "Welcome to Medicare" wellness exam.
6. Dr. Perez then asks Mrs. Crawford if she is having any signs or symptoms. She states that she feels pretty good most days, although she has noticed an increase in pain in her joints, especially her fingers. She is also having some issues with constipation. This is documented in the Review of Systems section. Click on the radio button next to sign/symptoms. **Yes** to indicate that the patient has that sign/symptom and **No** to indicate that they do not.
7. Click the **Save** button.

Height, weight, and blood pressure are documented in the Vital Signs section of SimChart for the Medical Office. Dr. Perez has asked you to document the following:

Height: 5 feet 6 inches
Weight: 175 pounds
Blood pressure: 136/72 right arm, sitting

---

1. While in the encounter from the previous task click on the **Record** drop-down menu and select **Vital Signs**.
2. From the **Vital Signs** tab click on the **Add** button (Fig. 8.3).
3. In the **Blood Pressure** section enter **136** in the **Systolic** field, **72** in the **Diastolic** field, select **Sitting** from the **Position** drop-down menu, select **Right arm** from the **Site** drop-down menu, and select **Manual with cuff** from the **Mode** drop-down menu. Click **Save**.
4. Click on the **Height/Weight** tab. Click on the **Add** button (Fig. 8.4).
5. In the **Height** section, enter **5** in the **ft** field and **6** in the **in** field.
6. In the **Weight** section, enter **175** in the **lb** field.
7. Click **Save**.

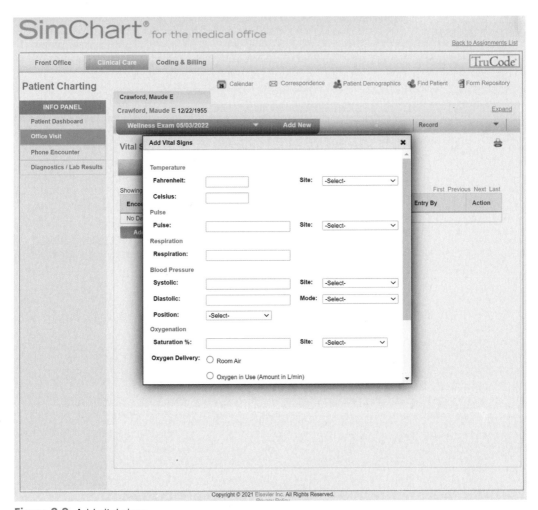

Figure 8.3 Add vital signs.

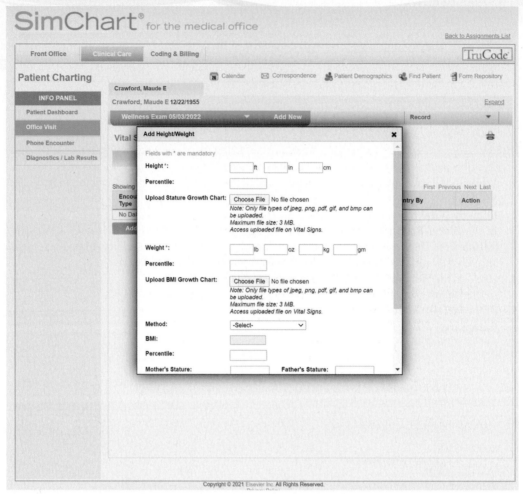

Figure 8.4 Add height/weight.

Another aspect covered in the "Welcome to Medicare" visit is reviewing prescription medications, over-the-counter medications, vitamins, and supplements. During this part of the visit with Mrs. Crawford she has indicated that she takes the following medications:

Simvastatin 1 tablet, 10 mg, daily
Lisinopril 1 tablet, 30 mg, daily
Levothyroxine 1 tablet, 25 mcg, daily
Calcium carbonate, 2 tablets, 600 mgs each, daily
Senior Multivitamin, 1 tablet daily

1. While in the encounter from the previous task click on the **Record** drop-down menu and select **Medications**.
2. From the **Prescription Medications** tab click the **Add Medication** button (Fig. 8.5).
3. From the **Medication** drop-down menu select **Simvastatin Tablet**.
4. From the **Strength** drop-down menu select **10**.
5. From the **Form** drop-down menu select **Tablet**.
6. From the **Route** drop-down menu select **Oral**.
7. From the **Frequency** drop-down menu select **Daily in the Evening**.
8. In the **Dose** field enter 1 tablet
9. In the **Status** section click on the **Active** radio button.
10. Click the **Save** button.

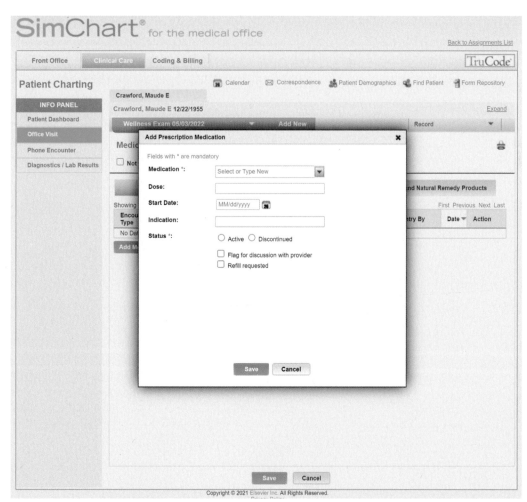

Figure 8.5 Add medications.

Day Eight

11. Use the same process to enter the lisinopril and levothyroxine.
12. To enter the calcium carbonate and Senior multivitamin click on the **Over-the-Counter Products** tab.
13. From the **Generic Name** drop-down menu select **Calcium Carbonate**.
14. From the **Form** drop-down menu select **Chewable Tablet**.
15. In the **Dose** field enter **2 tablets**.
16. In the **Frequency** field enter **Daily**.
17. From the **Route** drop-down menu select **Oral**.
18. In the **Strength** field enter 600 mgs.
19. In the **Status** section click on the **Active** radio button.
20. Click the **Save** button.
21. Use the same process to enter the Senior Multivitamin.

Another component of the "Welcome to Medicare" examination is a simple vision test. This done using a Snellen chart to test for distance visual acuity. Dr. Perez asks you to document the following results of Mrs. Crawford's Snellen exam:

> Right eye – 20/40
> Left eye – 20/20
> Both eyes – 20/20
> Wearing glasses

1. While in the encounter from the previous task click on the **Record** drop-down menu and select **Order Entry**.
2. Under **In-Office** click the **Add** button and select **Snellen Exam** from the **Order** drop-down menu (Fig. 8.6).
3. Enter the results of the exam in the appropriate fields.
4. Enter your name in the **Entry By** field.
5. Click on the **Save** button.

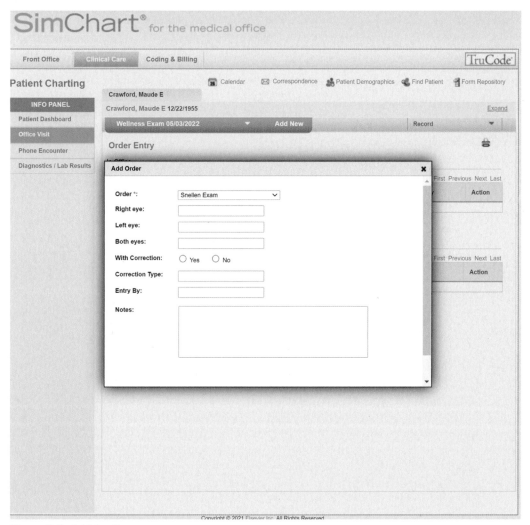

Figure 8.6 Add Snellen exam.

Task 8.10 Documenting Immunizations

For the last part of the "Welcome to Medicare" visit Dr. Perez reviews Mrs. Crawford's immunization history. Mrs. Crawford has brought documentation that she received the influenza and pneumococcal vaccines at the local public health clinic. Dr. Perez has asked you to document these vaccines:

> Influenza: IIV, 0.5 mL given in the right deltoid (IM) on 05/18/2022, no reaction
> Pneumococcal: Conjugate, 0.5 mL given in the left deltoid (IM) on 05/18/2022, no reaction

1. While in the encounter from the previous task click on the **Record** drop-down menu and select **Immunizations**.
2. Scroll down to locate **IIL, LAIV (Influenza/Flu)** and click on the green plus sign for #1 (Fig. 8.7).
3. Enter the information provided for the influenza vaccine. Click on the **Save** button.
4. Use the same process to enter the information for the pneumococcal vaccine.

Dr. Perez thanks you for your professionalism during this visit and your accurate documentation of Mrs. Crawford's "Welcome to Medicare" visit.

Only 2 days left in your practicum! Keep up the good work!

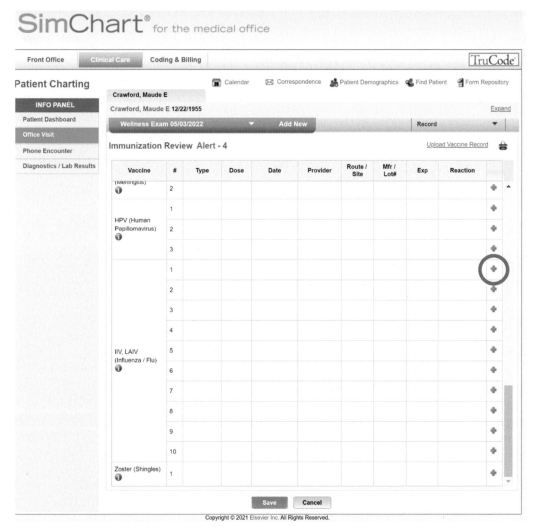

Figure 8.7 Add immunizations.

9. Day Nine

You are starting your ninth day in your practicum and Jill feels that you can work fairly independently. You will be working on tasks that you have done previously.

Your first task today is to schedule a new patient for an annual examination with Dr. Walden. Judy Merrill calls and requests an appointment on a Monday morning with Dr. Walden. In this situation you should use New Patient for the visit type and Annual Exam as the reason for the visit. Use the information below to schedule her appointment (refer to Box 1.1 for length of appointment).

Patient name: Judy M. Merrill
Date of birth: 05/21/1969
Insurance:
Aetna
1234 Insurance Way
Anytown, AL 12345
Phone: 800-123-2222
Policy holder: Judy Merrill
Social Security number: 322-88-3922
Policy/ID number: P78549S
Group number: 45789R

Schedule a New Patient Appointment

1. Open Dr. Walden's schedule and find the correct day and time.
2. Schedule the appointment for the appropriate amount of time (refer to Box 1.1 and Task 1.6).

You have asked Judy if she has time to give you the rest of her demographic information, and she has said yes, she does.

◎ PROFESSIONALISM

When working in a busy medical clinic, it is easy to get distracted. It is important to stay focused on the patient at all times, even when on the phone. By having your work station completely supplied with things like pens, scratch paper, clock, or watch, you can complete a phone call without having to search for a pen to write down a phone message. Patients can tell, even on the phone, if they do not have your complete attention. Eating, drinking, or chewing gum can all be sensed by the person on the other end of the phone call. You will have a much more satisfied patient if you make that phone call your priority.

Complete Demographic Informtion

Use the information below to complete the Patient Demographics section of the electronic health record for Judy Merrill.

Patient name: Judy M. Merrill
Date of birth: 05/21/1969
Address:
922 Old Farm Road
Anytown, AL 12345
Phone: 123-455-9246
Emergency contact: Pete Merrill
Emergency contact phone: 123-455-5823
Language: English
Race: White
Ethnicity: Not Hispanic or Latino
Employer: Anytown Law Firm
Insurance:
Aetna
1234 Insurance Way
Anytown, AL 12345
Phone: 800-123-2222
Policy holder: Judy Merrill
Social Security number: 322-88-3922
Policy/ID number: P78549S
Group number: 45789R

---

1. Click on the **Patient Demographics** icon and complete a **Patient Search**.
2. Enter all of the required information on the three tabs.

Task 9.2 Generating Appropriate Forms for a New Patient

As Judy is a new patient of the Walden-Martin Family Medical Clinic, you will need to send her all the forms required.

1. Using the **Correspondence** and **Form Repository** icons, complete the **New Patient Welcome** letter, **Notice of Privacy Practices**, **Patient Bill of Rights**, and the **Medical Records Release** (refer to Task 2.1).

2. **Save** all the documents to Judy's record.

To view the documents you have just created, click on the Find Patient icon and perform a Patient Search for Judy Merrill. You will land on the Patient Dashboard of the electronic health record. By scrolling down the page, you will see the New Patient Welcome letter in the correspondence section and the three forms you created in the Forms section. You can click on any of them to print them out if required by your instructor.

Task 9.3 Scheduling Appointments for Established Patients

Mrs. Burgel is calling to schedule a well-child visit for her daughter, Isabella Burgel, DOB 07/23/2019. Isabella is an established patient of Dr. Martin and her mother is requesting an appointment for next Thursday in the early afternoon.

Isabella Burgel

1. Find the appropriate date and time for this appointment on Dr. Martin's schedule and perform a **Patient Search** (refer to Task 1.3).
2. Add the appointment for the appropriate length of time to Dr. Martin's schedule (refer to Box 1.1).
3. Click the **Save** button.

Maude Crawford, DOB 12/22/1955, has also called to schedule an appointment for a recheck of her blood pressure. She is Dr. Martin's patient but has heard such good things about Jean Burke that she would like to see her for this visit.

 PROFESSIONALISM

Sometimes the smallest of gestures can make a patient's visit an exceptional visit. By saying please and thank you, and having a smile on your face, patients will feel like the clinic is a pleasant place to be and that you really care about them. It takes very little time on your part to be courteous and friendly, but it can make a big difference in how patients view their visits to the clinic.

Maude Crawford

1. Find the appropriate date and time for this appointment on Jean Burke's schedule and perform a **Patient Search**.
2. Add the appointment for the appropriate length of time to Jean Burke's schedule (refer to Box 1.1).
3. Click the **Save** button.

Task 9.4 Correcting Demographic Information

Patient demographic information can come to the medical office in several different ways. The patient may provide it directly or it may arrive from a different source, such as a returned letter from the U.S. Postal Service. Having the correct patient demographic information is key to billing correctly. Having accurate and complete demographic information allows for timely filing of claims and collection of insurance payments for the medical office. Jill has asked you to update the following patient's demographic information.

The statement that was mailed to Jana Green, DOB 05/01/1945, has been returned to the Walden-Martin Family Medical Clinic by the post office with a change of address label on it. It appears that Jana has moved into an apartment. Her new address is 851 University Drive, Apt 322, Anytown, AL 12345-1322.

1. Click on the **Patient Demographics** icon and perform a **Patient Search** (refer to Task 2.5).
2. Update the patient's address.
3. Click the **Save Patient** button.

When you make an appointment reminder phone call to Janine Butler, DOB 04/25/1977, you get a recorded message that states her phone number has changed to 123-492-2155.

1. Click on the **Patient Demographics** icon and perform a **Patient Search**.
2. Update the appropriate fields.
3. Click the **Save Patient** button.

Truong Tran, DOB 05/30/2000, has called the office to say that he has a new job at Anytown Fitness and also that his insurance information has changed (Fig. 9.1).

1. Click on the **Patient Demographics** icon and perform a **Patient Search**.
2. Update the appropriate fields.
3. Click the **Save Patient** button.

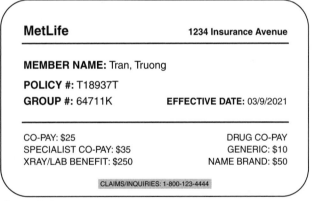

Figure 9.1 Truong Tran's insurance card.

Dr. Walden would like her patient Erma Willis, DOB 12/09/1956, to be seen by a neurosurgeon for issues related to worsening migraine symptoms. The neurosurgeon requested by Dr. Walden is Dr. Randall at Anytown Neurology Associates, 9075 Hillview Road, Anytown, AL 12345. She would like to refer Erma for five visits.

Diagnosis: Persistent migraine with aura, without cerebral infarction, intractable, without status migranosus; ICD-10 G43.519

Significant clinical information/symptoms: headache pain with aura for 3 weeks

Medications: Imitrex 50 mg

Walden-Martin Family Medical Clinic, phone 123-123-1234

Dr. Walden's NPI number: 987654321

---

1. Find the **Referral** form in the **Form Repository** and perform a **Patient Search**.
2. Using the information provided above, complete all necessary fields (refer to Task 3.3).
3. Click the **Save to Patient Record** button.

Mrs. Burgel has called back and says that she needs to reschedule Isabella's appointment for next week. She just found out that she will need to work on that day. She would like to schedule it for the following week on Wednesday in the early afternoon.

1. View Dr. Martin's schedule and find a time on Wednesday of the following week in the early afternoon that will work with Mrs. Burgel's schedule (refer to Task 1.2). Make a note of the date and time.
2. Locate Isabella Burgel's appointment on the calendar and click on it.
3. Click on the calendar icon next to the Date field and select the new date. If necessary, adjust the **Start Time** and **End Time** for the new appointment.
4. You will see a confirmation message. Click the **OK** button.

Tai Yan, DOB 4/7/1965, had a hysterectomy 6 weeks ago and her employer is asking for a certificate to return to work before she returns to her job full time. Dr. Perez has asked you to complete the form. Ms. Yan should be able to return to work on Monday of next week with no restrictions.

1. Click on the **Forms Repository** icon and locate the **Certificate to Return to Work or School** template (refer to Task 2.7).
2. Click on the **Patient Search** button at the bottom of the form and search for Tai Yan.
3. Complete the open fields with the information provided above.
4. Click the **Save to Patient Record** button.

Al Neviaser, DOB 06/21/1976, was recently seen in the emergency department of Anytown Hospital with acute pain on the left side, fever, and chills. A CT scan revealed that he had a cyst on his left kidney. Upon discharge from the hospital, he was referred to a nephrologist, Dr. Bean. He has a follow-up appointment with Dr. Bean in 2 weeks. Dr. Bean has requested that Mr. Neviaser have copies of previous x-rays sent to him for review before the appointment. Mr. Neviaser stops in at Walden-Martin to request that those x-rays be sent. Use the information below to complete the Medical Records Release form for Mr. Neviaser to sign so you can then send his records to his new provider. Remember that you are releasing the records from Walden-Martin Family Medical Clinic to the new provider.

New Provider:
Dr. Bean and Associates Nephrology Clinic
2020 Renal Drive
Anytown, AK 12345-1234
Phone: 555-579-1346
Fax: 555-579-2020
Expiration date: One year from today

---

1. Locate the **Medical Records Release** form and perform a **Patient Search** (Refer to Task 2.8).
2. Confirm the autopopulated information and complete the form for the x-ray/radiology records from Mr. Nevaiser's records from Walden-Martin Family Medical Clinic.
3. Click the **Save to Patient Record** button.

Julia Berkley, DOB 7/5/1998, is an established patient of Dr. Perez. Ms. Berkley is recently divorced and due to her multiple health issues, she would like her mother to have access to her health records and also to be able to talk to her doctors. A Disclosure Authorization form will need to be completed.

Peggy Gilbert
Address:
4173 1st Ave West
Anytown, AL 12345

---

1. Find the **Disclosure Authorization** in the **Form Repository** and perform a **Patient Search** (refer to Task 3.1).
2. Review the autopopulated fields and complete all other required fields.
3. Click the **Save to Patient Record** button.

The Disclosure Authorization has now been saved to Julia Berkley's record and can be used to give information to Peggy Gilbert when she requests it.

Megan Adams, DOB 9/27/1990, was recently seen by Dr. Walden for a sore throat, fever, and head-ache. Dr. Walden had ordered a rapid strep screen that came back negative. It is Walden-Martin's policy that if the rapid test comes back negative, a strep culture is done. Megan had asked that the results be emailed to her, as she would be unavailable by phone. The result of the strep culture is also negative, and Dr. Walden has asked you to send out the normal test results email.

1. Find the **Normal Test Results** template by clicking on the **Correspondence** icon, locating the template, and performing a **Patient Search** (refer to Task 4.1).
2. Review the autopopulated fields and complete all other required fields.
3. Click the **Send** button and a copy of the email will be saved to the patient record.

Jill is very impressed with your work today! You have completed all your tasks in a timely fashion. Keep up the good work! One more day to go!

10. Day Ten

◎ PROFESSIONALISM

As you complete your practicum, it is important to keep in mind those things that employers are looking for above and beyond knowledge of how a medical clinic works. During your practicum, your supervisors and mentors are also looking for enthusiasm and a positive attitude. These attributes go a long way toward making a team function well. They are also evaluating your work ethic. Did you take the initiative to find something to do when you had completed a given task? Did you ask what else you could do? Did you arrive on time every day or even a little early? Any practicum experience is a chance for you to show all aspects of yourself. It is very much an extended job interview, even if that organization is not hiring. You should be confident to ask anyone with whom you worked to be a reference, which will help you obtain a position in your chosen career.

Jill has asked that you work with Dr. Kahn as his scribe for one of his patients. You have worked with Dr. Kahn before and appreciate the opportunity to work with him on your last day.

Task 10.1 Documenting Chief Complaint, History of Present Illness, and Review of Systems

Tai Yan, DOB 4/7/1965, is being seen by Dr. Kahn regarding a dog bite she received earlier today. Dr. Kahn is examining the 4-cm laceration on her right palm. Ms. Yan states that the severity of the pain is 5 on a scale of 1 to 10, and describes the pain as throbbing and constant. Ibuprofen has helped the pain a little bit. During the review of systems, Ms. Yan denies fever, chills, sweats, and fatigue, but admits to joint swelling and injury. She reports no other signs and symptoms. Dr. Kahn asks you to document the chief complaint, history of the present illness, and the review of systems (refer to Task 2.9).

1. Click on the **Clinical Care** tab and locate Tai Yan's name in the List of Patients. Click on the radio button next to her name and then click on the **Select** button.
2. In order to enter the information into the EHR, you will need to create an encounter. Click on **Office Visit** in the Info Panel.
3. Select **Urgent Visit** for the Visit Type and **David Kahn, MD** for the Provider, and click on the **Save** button. At this time the medical record will open up and the **Record** drop-down menu will appear.
4. Click on **Chief Complaint** from the **Record** drop-down menu and document the chief complaint as described above, document the symptoms associated with the chief complaint in the **History of Present Illness** section. Within the **Review of Systems** section, select the **No** radio buttons for fever, chills, and fatigue; select the **Yes** radio buttons for joint swelling and injury.
5. Click the **Save** button.

Task 10.2 Documenting Vital Signs and Surgical History

Dr. Kahn asks you to document the following vital signs that were taken on Ms. Yan:

> Temperature – 99.1, tympanic
> Pulse – 96, regular, 2+
> Respiration – 14, regular, normal
> Blood Pressure – 124/86 left arm, sitting

While reviewing the patient's health history, Ms. Yan tells Dr. Kahn that she had an appendectomy 3 years ago at Anytown Hospital. Dr. Kahn asks you to document that in past surgeries.

1. From the **Vital Signs** tab, click on the **Add** button (refer to Task 8.7).
2. Document the vital signs listed above.
3. Click the **Save** button.
4. From the **Record** drop-down menu, select **Health History**.
5. Under **Past Surgeries**, click on the **Add New** button.
6. Enter a year from three years before today's date in **Date** field.
7. Enter **Anytown Hospital** in the **Location** field.
8. Enter **Appendectomy** in the **Type of Surgery** field.
9. Click the **Save** button.

An employee working the lab was injured when a bottle of chemical reagent was dropped, causing it to splash in their face and eyes. After a 15-minute eyewash and basic first aid, Dr. Perez assessed the employee and determined that no additional treatment was needed. Additional training on handling chemicals will be reviewed with the staff. Jill has asked that you complete the incident report for this accident (refer to Task 3.2).

1. Find the **Incident Form** in the **Form Repository**.
2. Complete all required fields. It is important to be specific and detailed in the documentation of an Incident Report.
3. Click the **Save** button.

Jill has discovered that Mora Siever, DOB 1/24/1972, has an outstanding balance on her account for audiometry that was performed on 4/25/2022. According to the explanation of benefits. This service is not covered by her insurance. Jill asks that you create the denial letter for Mora Siever (refer to Task 6.2).

1. Determine the balance on the account by viewing the **Ledger**.
2. Select the **Denial** letter template from the information panel on the left side of the screen and perform a **Patient Search**.
3. Verify the autopopulated information and enter the date of service, date of claim denial, the service that was denied, reason for denial, the outstanding balance, and the payment due date.
4. Click on the **Save to Patient Record** button.

Task 10.5 Creating a Prior Authorization Request

Two established patients of the Walden-Martin Family Medical Clinic need prior authorization for procedures. Jill has asked you to complete these requests.

Diego Lupez, DOB 08/01/1991, would like to have a vasectomy performed. Before scheduling the procedure, Dr. Martin has asked that you complete the Prior Authorization Request so that Diego can find out whether his insurance carrier will pay for the procedure.

1. Locate the **Prior Authorization Request** form and perform a **Patient Search** (refer to Task 4.6).
2. Use the information below to complete the form.

```
Ordering physician: James A. Martin
Provider contact name: Jill King
Place of service/treatment and address:
Walden-Martin Family Medical Clinic
1234 Anystreet
Anytown, AL 12345
Service requested: Vasectomy
Diagnosis/ICD code: ICD-10 Z98.52
Procedure/ CPT code: 55250
Injury related?: No
Workers' Compensation related: No
```

3. Click the **Save to Patient Record** button.

Celia Tapia, DOB 05/18/1979, needs to have an ingrown toenail removed. Celia is concerned that this may not be covered by her insurance. Dr. Martin has asked you to complete the Prior Authorization Request so that Celia knows before the procedure is scheduled whether her insurance carrier will pay for this procedure.

1. Locate the **Prior Authorization Request** form and perform a **Patient Search**.
2. Use the information below to complete the form.

```
Ordering physician: James A. Martin
Provider contact name: Jill King
Place of service/treatment and address:
Walden-Martin Family Medical Clinic
1234 Anystreet
Anytown, AL 12345
Service requested: Nail removal with matrix
Diagnosis/ICD code: Ingrowing nail;ICD-10 L60.0
Procedure/ CPT code: 11750
Injury related?: No
Workers' Compensation related: No
```

3. Click the **Save to Patient Record** button.

The Superbill for the wellness visit of Isabella Burgel, DOB 07/23/2019, needs to be completed. Use the information below and the fee schedule to complete the Superbill.

> Previous balance: $0.00
> Services provided: Established patient, well visit, 1-4 y
> Isabella's mother, Amanda Burgel, is the insured, ID number is WMF456987123, Group number is 65321B.
> Condition is not related to employment, auto accident, or other accident.
> Diagnosis: Routine child check; ICD-10 DZ00.129
> HIPAA form is on file. Date: Today's date

1. Click on the **Clinical Care** module and perform a search to locate Isabella Burgel, DOB 7/23/2019. Click on the radio button next to her name and then click on the **Select** button (refer to Task 3.6).
2. To create an encounter, click on **Office Visit** in the Info Panel. If encounters already exist for Isabella, you will need to click on the **Add New** tab.
3. Select **Wellness Exam** for the Visit Type and **James A. Martin, MD** for the Provider and click on the **Save** button.
4. After the encounter has been created, click on the **Coding and Billing** module and locate Isabella Bergel.
5. From the list of **Encounters Not Coded**, click on the one you created today. This will open up the Superbill.
6. Using the information provided above, complete the Superbill.
7. Click in the **I am ready to submit the Superbill** box, then click the **Yes** radio button in the **Signature on file** section and use today's date in the **Date** section.
8. Click the **Save** button and then click on the **Submit Superbill** button.

Task 10.7 Creating a Claim

The next step is to create a claim.

1. Click on **Claim** on the left side, perform a **Patient Search** if necessary, and you will see the encounter. Click on the paper and pencil icon to open the claim.
2. There are seven tabs for the claim. Review the autopopulated information for the five Patient Info, Provider Info, Payer Info, Encounter Notes, and Claim Info tabs. Add any missing information. Click the **Save** button for each tab.
3. On the **Charge Capture** tab, the **POS** (Place of Service) code can be found by clicking on the **Place of Service** link. Enter all necessary information. Click the **Save** button.
4. Click on the **Submission** tab and click the checkbox next to **I am ready to submit the Claim**.
5. Select the **Yes** radio button for **Signature on File** and enter today's date in the **Date** field.
6. Click the **Submit Claim** button.

Carl Bowden, DOB 4/5/1963, has sent in an application for life insurance so that the provider portion can be completed. You call Mr. Bowden to inform him that there is a $15.00 fee for this service, and Mr. Bowden agrees to have the form completed and be billed for the service. Document the charge for the fee in Mr. Bowden's ledger.

1. Click on the **Coding and Billing** tab and then select **Ledger** from the information panel on the left side of the screen. Perform a **Patient Search**.
2. Use today's date for the **Transaction Date** and **DOS**.
3. Enter Application fee for the service and 15.00 in the **Charges** column.
4. Click the **Save** button.

Because the fee for the completion of the life insurance application cannot be billed to Mr. Bowden's insurance, Jill has asked you to create a statement to be sent to Mr. Bowden for the balance of $15.00 (refer to Task 5.4)

1. Locate the **Patient Statement** in the **Form Repository** and perform a **Patient Search**.
2. Confirm the autopopulated fields.
3. Using today's date, complete the fields using **Application** for the description. The full charge will be the patient's responsibility and should be paid in full by 1 month from today.
4. Click the **Save to Patient Record** button.

Task 10.10 Completing the Day Sheet

Your last task is to complete the Day Sheet. Jill has asked that you enter the following services and payments on the Day Sheet for today:

Isabella Burgel: Services 99392 $75.00; old balance $346.00

Tai Yan: Services 99205 $119.00, 93000 $89.00; payment $10.00; old balance $0.00

Aaron Jackson: Services 99392 $75.00, 90471 $10.00, 90633 $33.00; old balance $0.00

Norma Washington: Services 99212 $32.00; payment $10.00; old balance $158.00

Anna Richardson: Services 99395 $80.00; old balance $35.00

Johnny Parker: Insurance payment (INSPYMT) $137.30; adjustment $12.23; old balance $137.30

Walter Biller: Insurance payment (INSPYMT) $157.90; adjustment $35.00: old balance $820.00

Day Sheet Entries

Using one line for each patient, post the CPT codes in the Service column and use the code INSPYMT for insurance payments in the Service column. You will have to calculate the new balance by starting with the old balance, adding any charges, and subtracting any payments and/or adjustments.

1. Click on the **Coding and Billing** tab to locate the **Day Sheet** on the left side.
2. Using the information provided above, enter all of the charges, payments, and adjustments for each patient on a separate line, using the **Add Row** button as needed.

Daily Proof of Posting; Accounts Receivable Proof

To verify that all of the numbers have been entered correctly, you will need to complete the Daily Posting Proof. The Accounts Receivable Proof provides the accounts receivable balance after the day's activities. This amount is carried forward to the next day's Day Sheet.

1. Using the column totals that have been autocalculated, complete the **Daily Posting Proof**. Your final total should match the total in Column D. If not, you will need to recheck the numbers entered into the Day Sheet. Make sure that your math is correct when adding the fees entered in the Charges column and calculating the New Balance.
2. Complete the **Accounts Receivable Proof**.

  You have completed the last task for the practicum! You have impressed Jill and all of the providers at the Walden-Martin Family Medical Clinic with your attention to detail and ability to stay on task. The skills you have learned while at the clinic will serve you well in your chosen career.

  Congratulations!

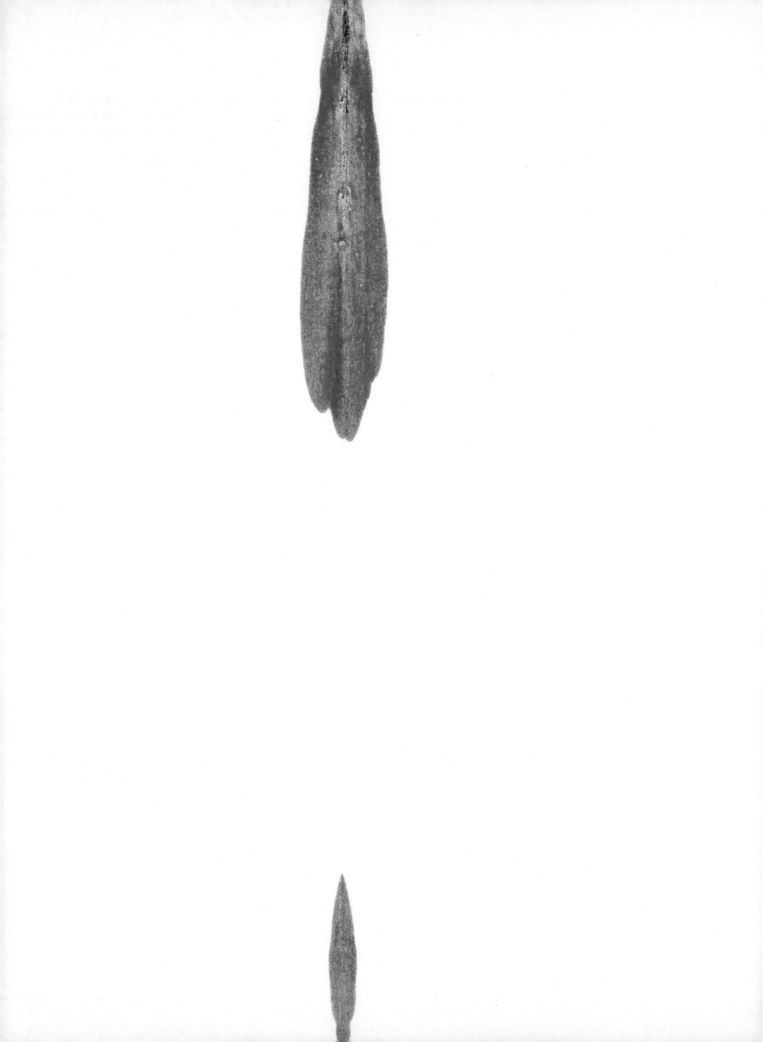